THE CHIEF: DOCTOR WILLIAM OSLER

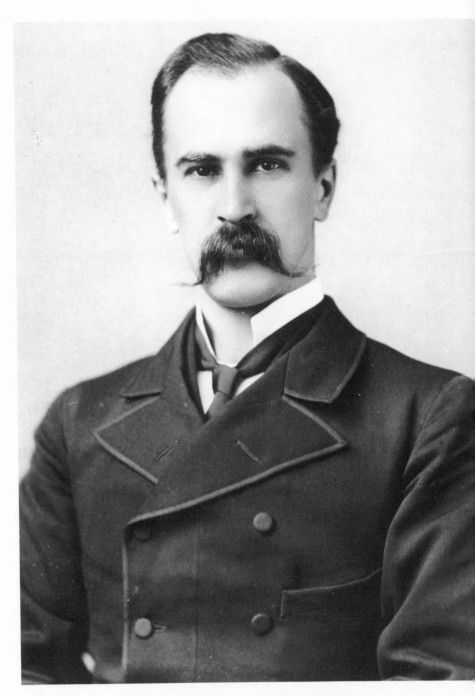

William Osler, October 29, 1881

The Chief:

DOCTOR WILLIAM OSLER

R. Palmer Howard

SCIENCE HISTORY PUBLICATIONS

U.S.A.

To the memory of Campbell and Ottilie Howard, Thomas and Marjorie Futcher, and all who shared the affectionate guidance of William and Grace Osler.

First published in the United States by
Science History Publications, U.S.A
a division of
Watson Publishing International
Post Office Box 493, Canton, MA 02021
© R. Palmer Howard 1983
Printed and manufactured in the U.S.A.

Published with the aid of grants from The Friends of The University of Iowa Libraries, Iowa City, and the John P. McGovern Foundation, Houston, Texas

Library of Congress Cataloging in Publication Data

Howard, R. Palmer, 1912–
  The chief, Doctor William Osler.

  Includes bibliographical references and index.
  1. Osler, William, Sir, 1849–1919.   2. Physicians—
Canada—Biography.   3. Physicians—Canada—Correspon-
dence.   I. Title.
R464.08H69 1983   610'.92'4   83–20234
ISBN 0–88135–000–1

Contents

Figures and Illustrations

Illustrations were prepared from originals in the Howard or Futcher family Collections unless otherwise indicated.

Prefatory Note

FIVE YEARS AGO, on a brief visit to the University of Oklahoma Health Sciences Center, I was privileged to be shown some letters and photographs relating William Osler to the Howard families and friends. These interesting materials belong to R. Palmer Howard, M.D., a vigorous and scholarly grandson of one of Osler's colleagues. The first R. Palmer Howard was Professor and later Dean of Medicine at McGill College in Montreal.

The text was prepared using eighty-three letters from William Osler to Campbell and Ottilie Howard, a similar number to Campbell Howard's sister, Marjorie (the late Mrs. T. B. Futcher), a letter to A. S. Warthin, Osler correspondence with Principal Peterson of McGill University and miscellaneous documents in the McGill and University of Iowa Archives. Also included are fifty photographs of the Osler and Howard families, and other Osler friends. Less than ten of the photographs have been published previously. Largely based on these documents, the author has prepared a marvelous account of the close relationship of William Osler to the Palmer Howard family. He also carefully reviews other highlights of Osler's remarkable career.

The author's essay briefly summarizes Osler's career as a distinguished physician-educator and includes a most intimate account of the Osler-Howard interactions beginning in Montreal and continuing until Osler's death in 1919. The senior Doctor Howard was among the earliest to recognize Osler's genius; first, when he taught him as a medical student and later, even more clearly, when they served as fellow physicians at the McGill Medical School and the Montreal General Hospital.

The absence of any hint of jealousy and competition between

these two extraordinary physicians is as notable as the clear evidence of the reinforcement each gave the other during their distinguished careers. The letters reflect Osler's interest in advancing the professional careers of young physicians, while acting as a family confidant and affectionate counselor.

The text includes also a brief, but interesting, account of Mrs. Osler's relationship to the Howard family. One is impressed that William Osler made a special effort to keep in touch with Palmer Howard's children after the death of their mother. The influence of Osler particularly on Campbell Howard covered the period of his medical training in Europe, and probably influenced his appointment as Professor and Chairman of the Department of Medicine at the University of Iowa. There are rich biographical vignettes of other family members; the most sparse account is of the author, undoubtedly related to his modesty.

A short epilogue reviews the distinguished career of Campbell Howard, the author's father, who was Osler's godson. Bibliophiles and Oslerians will find the biographical notes and tabulation of important dates in the lives of the Osler and Howard families a useful adjunct to the references.

Students of Osler and physicians and historians generally will find that the letters and photographs serve as insightful illustrations of Osler's humanism. They will also be reminded that Osler had the knack of choosing his friends carefully and cultivating them over long periods of time. The reader will be stimulated to return to Cushing's *The Life of Sir William Osler* to appreciate how much of Osler's character has been revealed through this small, but remarkable, collection of letters. The author has succeeded in writing a scholarly essay without being emotionally influenced unduly by his close relationship with the Howard family.

Martin M. Cummings, M.D.

June 21, 1983

Introduction

WILLIAM OSLER had a great impact on my grandfathers, the physicians R. Palmer Howard of Montreal and Henry P. Wright of Ottawa, Canada, and his influence extended to their children. During my own professional experience in medicine, an interest in history was an avocation until 1965 when Stewart Wolf, Professor of Medicine at Oklahoma University, facilitated the opportunity for me to develop a program in the history of medicine.

Subsequently I received a few Osler letters to the senior Palmer Howard, and eighty-three others, almost all from William Osler to my father, Campbell P. Howard. I have also inherited books, portraits, and other artifacts, along with many informal photographs of the Osler family taken by my mother while she was in Oxford during 1909–1911 and later.

Following my first presentation based on these materials at the American Osler Society Meeting in May, 1978, I sought Osleriana from other family members. I am most grateful to my cousins, Palmer Howard Futcher, Gwendolen Futcher and Grace Norsworthy, for allowing me to select from ninety-four letters from William Osler to their mother, Marjorie (Howard) Futcher, and from her photographs. These previously unpublished items constitute a valuable addition to Osler biography, and contain some important evidence of the chain of influence from the senior Palmer Howard to William Osler, and from Osler to his pupils Campbell P. Howard and Thomas B. Futcher. It is unfortunate that other letters from Osler to Thomas Futcher were destroyed. Osler's letters to R. Jared B. Howard, Muriel (Howard) Eberts and their families have also apparently been destroyed, with a single exception in the Marjorie Futcher collection.

I also thank Thomas A. Warthin for allowing me to cite a letter written in 1916 by Osler to his father, Professor Alfred S. Warthin. Colin K. Russel, Marion Wright, and Mrs. John Fulton kindly contributed photographs for this publication.

The McGill University Archives contain the outgoing and incoming correspondence (1895–1919) of Principal Sir William Peterson. There were identified eighteen letters from Osler and twenty-five to Osler, as well as relevant correspondence with Lord Strathcona, Campbell Howard and others. The University Archives, Special Collections, University of Iowa Libraries, hold valuable correspondence and minutes relative to the College of Medicine from the period of Abraham Flexner's visit in 1909 through C.P. Howard's tenure. Prints were identified or obtained from the negatives in the Notman Photographic Archives, McCord Museum, McGill University. I am indebted to the staffs of the aforementioned repositories for their assistance.

Among many who supplied information about subjects mentioned in the Osler correspondence, I am specially grateful to Margaret A. Revere, A.H.T. Robb-Smith, Sir Richard Doll, Thomas E. Keys, Marion Wright, Muriel (Howard) Douglas, Barnaby J. Howard, the late Edith Lady Congleton, Beatrice (Eberts) Price, Alan and Marion Gibbons.

Courteous service was rendered by the library staffs of the College of Physicians of Philadelphia, University of Kansas College of Health Sciences and Hospital, Yale School of Medicine, Duke University Medical Center, Mayo Foundation, Bodleian Library, Royal College of Physicians, Wellcome Institute for the History of Medicine, National Library of Medicine, Directorate of History of the Canadian National Defense Headquarters, University of Oklahoma and Health Sciences Center, State Library of Iowa, University of Iowa Libraries, and McGill University Libraries, including the Medical Library and Osler Library of The History of Medicine.

For my training in history and related fields, I thank John Duffy, Robert E. Bell, the late Walter Rundell, Jr., Donald Berthrong and Duane H.D. Roller. For other professional support, I acknowledge especially Lloyd G. Stevenson, Mark R. Johnson, the late Robert M. Bird, Leonard M. Eddy, Virginia E. Allen, Robert E. Rakel, John P.McGovern, Charles G. Roland and others of The American Osler Society. For secretarial and typing assistance, I am most grateful to Phyllis Randolph, Bobbie Antrim, Erma McKee, Pat Cassabaum and Helen Haugan. The Department of Family

Practice, University of Iowa Hospitals and Clinics, provided me with important support in completing this book.

In conclusion, I sincerely acknowledge John Duffy, Palmer Futcher, H. Wayne Morgan, William B. Bean and Edward H. Bensley for their advice in the composition of my manuscript, and my wife, Muriel, for her help in many ways.

CHAPTER I

Early Years in Canada

WILLIAM OSLER was born in 1849 in a cabin at Bond Head, Ontario, on the edge of the virgin forest, about forty miles north of Toronto, Canada. His father was an Anglican (here, called Episcopalian) missionary clergyman and his mother was an understanding and resolute woman. After marrying in 1837 in Falmouth, Cornwall, they arrived in the new pioneer settlement soon after it had been surveyed. They had seven children before the youngest boy was born. He was named William because on that day the Irish villagers were celebrating the Battle of the Boyne in which William of Orange's Protestant forces gained a victory.

When William was eight years old, his father accepted a parish church in Dundas, a settled town near the present city of Hamilton, Ontario. William grew up to be a bright, athletic boy. He was a leader among his friends in mischievous behavior at Barrie School, which he entered when he was fifteen years of age in October, 1864.

In January 1866, he transferred to a new school at Weston. Its founder and warden had arranged that it be affiliated with an Anglican Church college and thus it was named Trinity College School. Osler's parents hoped he would learn music and cultural graces in preparation for becoming a clergyman. On the other hand, William was inspired by the warden, the Reverend William Johnson, to the study of nature. He enjoyed collecting on the field trips, mounting specimens and using the microscope. In the 1860s, very few people in America were familiar with this instrument, and its use was not taught to medical students. While under the broad cultural influence of the school, Osler acquired a one-volume Shakespeare and a recent edition of Sir Thomas Browne's

Religio Medici (1642), both of which influenced him deeply. Browne's philosophy, a blending of scholarly contemplation about nature and mankind with a simple Christian faith, became Osler's support along "the way of life". William concentrated on his class assignments sufficiently to graduate at the head of the school in June, 1867.

William Osler entered Trinity College in Toronto in the autumn of 1867 with the intent of becoming a clergyman like his father. However, he continued to pursue his interests in biology with Mr. Johnson and his friend, Dr. James Bovell.

Osler spent only one year at Trinity College in the Arts Program. Since none of his four elder brothers selected their father's profession, William Osler surely disappointed his parents by wishing to study medicine, but they understandingly accepted his decision. He entered the Toronto Medical School in October 1868 and, under the fatherly tutelage of Doctor Bovell, applied himself industriously to the preclinical subjects for two years. Bovell's life served as a warning as well as a model. He lacked organization and punctuality, and dissipated his energies through attempts to interpret the mysteries of life simultaneously from scientific and religious viewpoints. Yet, he stimulated his pupil in the available laboratory methods and, at the same time, influenced him to read widely from the great books of science and literature. Though Osler avoided his teacher's pitfalls, Bovell's influence was powerful and enduring. When Bovell was planning to leave Toronto for the West Indies, he recommended that Osler transfer for the fall session of 1870 to the older and more renowned McGill Medical School. McGill, in Montreal, which was the largest Canadian city at the time, had better clinical facilities.

Osler had already published his first scientific paper, *Christmas and the Microscope,* in which he described the *infusoria* and other microscopic species in a country spring near his home. Though the Toronto school provided no courses in histology, Osler observed the cysts of *trichina spiralis* in one of his anatomy subjects. With such a background, he was uniquely prepared to enter clinical training at McGill.

At the age of twenty-one, William Osler had a fine personality and enjoyed nature studies and the company of people younger or older than himself. Although he did not always get A's in his classwork, he enjoyed reading deeply and widely. The McGill Medical Library had limited holdings. A better collection was in the home of the Professor of Medicine, Robert Palmer Howard.

Osler's first roommate in Montreal was a medical student, Henry Wright, who was a cousin of Doctor Howard. After Wright introduced him to the Professor, Osler visited Howard's library freely in the evenings to read the German, French and English medical journals. He often browsed to late hours, with the Professor, seeking more detailed information from his fine collection of reference books. Howard had studied under Graves and Stokes in Dublin, and elsewhere in Britain and France. The McGill medical teachers provided excellent bedside instruction, and made clinical clerking a serious business.[1]

Doctor Palmer Howard was appointed Dean of Medicine in 1882. While maintaining a busy general practice, he was always an active teacher, and was considered an expert in internal medicine throughout Canada and the United States.[2]During one session he examined all patients with lung lesions in the Montreal General Hospital because the experiments of J.A. Villemin in 1868 had demonstrated that the poison of the tuberculous lesion was specific and inoculable. This was about fourteen years before Robert Koch identified the tubercule bacillus. At this earlier time, however, Howard wished to compare the clinical findings by Laennec's method with the postmortem examinations which each attending physician performed.

Howard was immediately attracted by the curiosity and industry of the young William Osler, whose special ability with the microscope provided information to supplement the studies of both student and professor. William Osler graduated in 1872 with a prize for his final thesis, which was illustrated by many microscopic specimens.

Osler went abroad for two years postgraduate education. He spent the first year in Britain. While working in the laboratory of Professor Burdon-Sanderson at University College, London, Olser made a significant scientific contribution; he discovered the third type of blood corpuscle, the platelet. Osler visited many British hospitals and clinics to study other aspects of physiology and general medicine, including surgery, neurology, dermatology and other branches. After October 1873, Osler visited medical centers on the European Continent. He was inspired by the pathologist, Rudolf Virchow, in Berlin. He also visited prominent internists and specialists in Berlin and Vienna. In each of those cities he remained for four or five months, also spending a short time in Paris. The McGill faculty wished to have the bright young Osler back in Montreal, but he turned down their first offer to teach medical botany, which he was not then studying. After completing his report on the blood platelets, for presentation by Burdon-Sanderson before the Royal Society in London on June 18, 1874, Osler sailed home, his future undecided.

In July 1874, Doctor Howard wrote that Professor J. Morley Drake had resigned for health reasons, and he offered Osler the vacancy as Lecturer of the Institutes of Medicine. Osler accepted this offer, performed well and the following year, when just twenty-six years old, he was promoted to Professor. The Edinburgh University term "institutes" meant the beginning or fundamental principles of the discipline. Osler taught physiology and pathology, and later added a course in histology.

From 1874 to 1884, Osler progressed in the medical college and community. In 1875, he volunteered to attend the smallpox isolation ward of the Montreal General Hospital. This was an unpopular and dangerous task. Usually the senior attending physicians supervised this ward in rotation for three month periods. This opportunity increased the availability of postmortem material for Osler, initiating his extensive pathological and clinical reports. As a consequence of good service in the volunteer capacity for about eight months, Osler was paid $600 for continuing to serve until a separate smallpox hospital was opened by the city early in 1876. Most of his remuneration was used for a previous obligation; he had ordered fifteen microscopes from France for the twelve students in his new class in histology. His annual professorial salary was less than $1,000 and private practice income provided only a few hundred dollars, earned mostly from house visits or office calls in Dr. Howard's absence.

During the 1876 summer session through July, Osler was busy teaching both clinical microscopy and postmortem demonstrations at the McGill-associated Montreal General Hospital, where he had been appointed pathologist. The exacting pathological duties and preparations for the classes apparently delayed the completion of obligations undertaken for his preceptor and his own literary activities. Palmer Howard wrote the "Canada Report" for the first (1875) international review of chest diseases under the direction of Horace Dobell. Osler had agreed to write the section in place of Howard for the 1876 volume but the deadline for this task was rapidly approaching. Osler was also gathering information to assist his elder friend to improve the regulations for licensure in Quebec, and to establish a uniform practice act throughout

Canada; the latter effort, unfortunately, was premature, but finally achieved in 1912 by Thomas Roddick.

The close association between the older and younger teacher-physicians is well borne out by Osler's letter written at the beginning of August 1876 to Howard, who was presumably at the family summer home on the St. Lawrence shore: "I hope the Medical Register with Act arrived safely. You should have had the enclosed report earlier but I have been kept away from all such work and cannot even get an hour for reading. The consequence is my paper on haemorrhagic Small-pox must remain over as I have not quite finished it. I was in Brantford a few days last week helping Dr. [James] Kerr get married."(3)

"That report for Dr. Dobell is due about the end of August. I have the no's of the Journals for the past year by me and will make it out & submit it to you before the middle of the month."(4)

In 1878, when only twenty-eight years of age, William Osler's industry and reputation resulted in his nomination and election to the coveted position of Attending Physician at the Montreal General Hospital. The originality and vitality he had previously demonstrated in the laboratory were now evident in the clinical setting. In the words of a contemporary witness: "When therefore his time came to take charge of a section of the hospital, older doctors looked on with bated breath, expecting disastrous consequences. He began by clearing up his ward completely. All the unnecessary semblances of sickness and treatment were removed; it was turned from a sick-room into a bright, cheerful room of repose. Then he started in with his patients. Very little medicine was given. To the astonishment of everyone, the chronic beds, instead of being emptied by disaster, were emptied rapidly through recovery; under his stimulating and encouraging influence the old cases nearly all disappeared, the new cases stayed but a short time. The revolution was wonderful. It was one of the most forceful lessons in treatment that had ever been demonstrated."(5)

During a decade on the McGill faculty Osler wrote many articles; among them were pieces on trichinosis and on congenital and acquired lesions of the heart, drawing from his pathological experience at the Montreal General Hospital and the Veterinary College. His articles on clinical topics were also published frequently in the Canadian, American and British Journals. With his energy and personal qualities, he stimulated his young col-

leagues and the older members of the faculty to increased participation in the local and national medical meetings, and to prepare articles for publication. His inspiration was clearly enun-
ciated in 1880 by Howard in the opening paragraphs of his
article, "Cases of Leucocythemia."[6]

When in October 1882 Dean Howard delivered the main address at the Semi-Centennial Celebration of the McGill Medical
College, Osler was secretary of the Faculty. After summarizing its
history, Howard mentioned the progress under Principal J. William Dawson. He then reported the first employment of the microscope in student teaching, during 1875, and other important
advances by "the indefatigable Professor of Institutes", such as
demonstrations in morbid anatomy. He stressed the need for a
larger museum, more apparatus for teaching, and the appointment of additional faculty for the instruction of small groups of
students at the beside, all matters in which Osler would be participating.[7]

During the summer of 1878, Osler had passed the examination
for membership in the Royal College of Physicians of London. In
1883, immediately after the minimal five year lapse, he was ele-
vated to fellowship in the Royal College in recognition of his
numerous publications and frequent attendance at professional
meetings in Canada, the United States, and Britain, one of the
youngest Canadians ever to have received this honor. Although
his career as Professor and consulting physician at the McGill
Medical School was now assured, he was soon to consider leaving
for an opportunity in a more prestigious center.

During 1884, the Professor of the Practice of Medicine at the
University of Pennsylvania, Alfred Stillé, resigned because of age,
and William Pepper was promoted to succeed him. This left a
vacancy in the junior professorship which would presumably be
filled by another candidate from Philadelphia. William Osler was
already serving on the editorial board of *The Medical News* published in that city. Through his visits and attendance at medical
meetings in the United States he was well known to several leading Philadelphia physicians, including S. Weir Mitchell. Accordingly, Professor H.C. Wood travelled to Montreal in June, 1884. He
returned with a glowing report. William Osler, however, provided
another account of his eventual selection. He was abroad when
Dr. S.W. Mitchell and his wife arranged a dinner engagement in
London later that summer. Cherry pie was served, and Osler
passed the test by disposing of the stones in a genteel manner.

The McGill medical faculty endeavored to keep Osler in Montreal. Dean Palmer Howard wrote that the Faculty Board would establish a separate chair of "Pathology and Comparative Pathology", and increase Osler's professorial salary to $1,600 a year. Howard continued with a sincere statement of his great value to McGill: ". . . not only on account of your abilities as a teacher, your industry and enthusiasm as a worker, your personal qualities as a gentleman, a colleague and a friend; not only on account of the work you have already done in and for the school, but also because of the capabilities we recognize in you for future useful work, both in original investigation, which shall add reputation to McGill, and in systematic teaching of any of the branches of Medical Science you may care to cultivate; and finally because we have for years felt that vitalizing influence upon us individually exercised by personal contact with you—analogous to that produced by a potent ferment."[8] Osler, however, had made his decision. In October, 1884, he arrived in Philadelphia to fill the Chair of Clinical Professor of Medicine at the University of Pennsylvania, the position he held for the next five years.

CHAPTER II

Osler at Philadelphia and Baltimore

AT PENNSYLVANIA, William Pepper, the incumbent Professor of the Practice of Medicine and his predecessor, Alfred Stillé, were excellent orators and talented at delivering formal lectures on medicine to the students. Osler was not so gifted in oratory, and was less formal in his attire and manner than other Philadelphia professors. He preferred to teach his students in small groups, working directly from the clinical manifestations in each patient. This method of bedside teaching had come from Leyden, through pupils of Boerhaave, to the Edinburgh Medical School, and thence to Philadelphia with Morgan, Shippen and Rush. It had also been carried from Edinburgh, by the founding professors of McGill Medical College, to Montreal where it persisted during Osler's student days.

Osler devoted himself to student teaching, participation in medical societies and writing rather than to private practice. He spent considerable time with clinic patients at the University Hospital and the Philadelphia Hospital or "Blockley." When his friend, S. Weir Mitchell, appreciated his interest, Osler also attended the Philadelphia Orthopedic Hospital and Infirmary for Nervous Diseases. At this institution his careful studies resulted in many articles on nervous disorders in children. In re-examinations of 110 patients more than two years after attacks of chorea, he demonstrated the presence of organic valvular heart disease in forty-three patients, and doubtful or "functional" murmurs in eleven others. A history of articular rheumatism coincided in a minority of the subjects with endocarditis complicating chorea.[9] Osler also stimulated the younger physicians and students to perform clinical laboratory studies and research. When Charles Laveran reported the protozoa in the red blood cells of malaria, Osler was not only skeptical, but at first unable to accept the evidence. After many months of tireless effort, however, he convinced himself, and was the first in America to publish confirmation of Laveran's discovery.[10]

His contributions to *The Medical News* and other journals comprised numerous original studies and carefully selected and thoughtful reviews on a wide range of medical literature. He participated actively in the pathological, neurological, biological and other medical societies, notably the College of Physicians of Philadelphia. Osler gained the friendship and esteem of the elder leaders, and the devoted admiration of the younger men. Among his students and colleagues, he infused the love of the classics and professional literature. He continued his interest and donations to the Library of the College of Physicians throughout his life.

William Osler by no means neglected his former professional associations or missed opportunities to make new ones while a resident of Philadelphia. Early in 1885 he delivered the Gulstonian lectures at the Royal College of Physicians in London on "Malignant Endocarditis". These were highly original and warmly received.[11] A London instrument maker then constructed for him a binaural stethoscope which medical students used in place of the monaural models.

In the autumn of 1885, William Pepper, James Tyson, and Osler, of Philadelphia, R.T. Edes of Boston, and Francis Delafield and others of New York were among the organizers of the Association of American Physicians. Soon augmented by Palmer Howard of Montreal and other physicians from New York and Boston, they came to be recognized as the founders of the well-known association. Osler probably nominated his friend Palmer Howard as one of the guests to be inducted as Honorary Fellows at the Centennial Celebration of the College of Physicians in Philadelphia on January 3, 1887. Weir Mitchell gave the commemorative address on the history of medicine in Philadelphia. This address was published in the *Medical News* along with Osler's editorial comments.[12] Already having a sound foundation in physiology and pathology, Osler achieved professional maturity in Philadelphia. He gained from further association with talented physicians in a large hospital center and he showed himself to be a gifted and inspiring teacher at the bedside of the patient.[13]

The reputation of Osler's invigorating spirit spread from Philadelphia to the medical men in other American cities. In October, 1888, John Shaw Billings and William H. Welch nominated Osler for the appointment of Physician-in-Chief at the new, but unfinished, Johns Hopkins Hospital in Baltimore. He continued his activities in Philadelphia vigorously during the intervening six months. Among Osler's many friends in Philadelphia were S. Weir Mitchell, J. William White, James Wilson, and Samuel W. Gross and his wife, the former Grace Revere. In March and April, 1889, attacks of pneumonia claimed two of Osler's intimate friends. Although he was attended by Osler and other clinicians, S. W. Gross died. He requested his colleague's continued friendship for Grace. [14]

Osler's teacher and supporter in Montreal, Palmer Howard, died on March 28, 1889. Howard's first wife, Mary Frances Chipman, had died in September, 1872 shortly after William Osler graduated from McGill Medical School. Their only son, Jared, later entered medical school and won a prize for excellence in Osler's clinical and laboratory courses. He also gained the Holmes Gold Medal for highest overall standing on graduation in 1882. He studied abroad for two years, attained the F.R.C.S. in England, and was appointed demonstrator in anatomy at McGill and assistant surgeon at the Montreal General Hospital in 1884. In 1888, he married Margaret Charlotte, only child of Sir Donald Smith. After 1896, Jared Howard and his family lived in London, and his father-in-law was appointed High Commissioner for Canada and created Baron Strathcona and Mount Royal. Lord Strathcona began his donations to McGill University, especially the medical school and affiliated hospitals, during Palmer Howard's lifetime and continued them later. He also answered many appeals from Osler and others for the support of academic and medical causes in Great Britain.[15]

On June 10, 1874, Palmer Howard married Emily Severs, his second wife. Thus, Osler's appointment at McGill as Lecturer, later Professor, of the Institutes, soon brought him the mutual affection of the second Mrs. Howard, and her children, Muriel, Campbell, Bruce, and Marjorie. The parents chose William Osler as a godfather for Campbell. In 1882, before von Behring's specific antitoxin was discovered in Germany, Bruce died of diphtheria.

Though William Osler was in Philadelphia, he frequently saw Palmer Howard and his family, and he returned to Montreal immediately on learning of his friend's grave illness. He not only comforted his wife, Emily, but led the three younger children to their father's bedside and continued to hold a special affection for them thereafter. Osler's high regard for Palmer Howard as a man and physician is recorded in "The Student Life", the notice of death, and formal obituary.[16] Emily Howard retained many tributes to her husband from the daily newspapers and letters. She undoubtedly appreciated the words of McGill's famous Principal, Sir William Dawson: ". . . I cannot trust myself to say anything of the friend who has gone from us for the present. I feel too much depressed by the loss sustained in the public interests with which he was identified, and in which I had the privilege on some occasions of working with him."[17]

William Osler kept in touch with the widow and young children of Palmer Howard. He sent his godson Campbell a picture postcard of the Eiffel Tower purchased in June, 1890 during his tour of the European medical centers. Osler's affectionate wishes for the family health were not fulfilled. Emily Howard died from breast cancer, at the age of fifty-two, on June 9, 1892.

At the time of their mother's death, Muriel was seventeen, Campbell fifteen, and Marjorie only ten years old. With adequate inheritance, they lived with several relatives in Montreal, while Muriel and Campbell completed their education. "Docie O" and his affectionate wife, "Aunt Grace" Osler, watched over them by exchange of visits and letters as if they were their own children. Always one of Osler's favorites, Muriel established herself readily in Montreal. In 1904 she married Edmond M. Eberts, M.D., surgeon at the Montreal General Hospital. They had five children, but soon after the last was born, she died on May 31, 1913.

The younger Howard children, Campbell, and especially Marjorie, had few recollections of their father. From their earliest memories, the figure of "Docie O" stood clear as a playmate— amusing, wise and comforting. By his visits and letters, he showed his affection for them with constancy. With some reserve, Campbell, and more openly Marjorie, came to regard him in the role of father.

Campbell attended Montreal High School before spending three years in the McGill College of Arts. He performed conspicuously on the football team and was a leader in the college fraternal and social activities. After successfully completing the requirements for the B.A. degree in 1897, Osler wrote on September 16 as Campbell entered the medical School: "Just a line to wish you good luck & God-speed in your medical work. The hopes of all of your father's dear friends are set on you. I know you will work steadily & surely. Let me know of any of your troubles & worries. I should like to stand to you in the same relation your father did to me. I can never repay what he did in the way of example & encouragement. Aunt Grace [Osler] is not yet back. I am going to Boston tonight to see her."[18]

This letter reveals several important and characteristic traits of William Osler. In addition to offering Campbell his father as a successful model, he stressed the need for steady work from the beginning in order to reach his professional goal, a theme he expanded in a later brilliant address to the entering medical students at the University of Toronto.[19]

Shortly before Campbell began the second year at the McGill Medical College, he received a book which he forever prized. W. Osler, *The Principles and Practice of Medicine*, 3rd edition, 1898, was inscribed: "Campbell Howard, with the author's love, Aug. 26, 1898". Campbell devoted himself assiduously to his medical courses and graduated in June 1901. He then began a year of internship at the Montreal General Hospital.

While the children of Palmer Howard were growing up, Osler's career continued its distinguished progress at the Johns Hopkins Medical Institutions.[20] The personal and professional development of William Osler took place at an opportune time. Johns Hopkins had provided separate charters for the University and Hospital, and the founder selected highly capable and qualified men for their boards of trustees. The first president of the University, Daniel Coit Gilman, was appointed in 1874. He succeeded in his aim to select the best available men without regard to their location or nationality. While becoming famous as the Director of the Surgeon-General's Library in Washington, John Shaw Billings submitted the plans and supervised the construction of the Johns Hopkins Hospital. He also provided the ideals for the medical college and gave lectures on medical history, education and jurisprudence. Billings interviewed William H. Welch and supported the Berlin Professor Julius Cohnheim's recommendation to appoint him to be Professor of Pathology in 1884.

Welch had trained under Cohnheim, Ludwig and other leading scientists in Germany, returning to New York City in 1878. There he established a pathological laboratory at the Bellevue Hospital Medical College, which was successful, despite little financial support. In 1885 Welch studied the latest bacteriological and pathological advances abroad and in 1886, at the age of thirty-six, he began work in Baltimore. Gilman, Billings, and Welch were chiefly responsible for selecting additional faculty and staff for the Hopkins Medical Institutions. Welch served as Chairman of the Hospital Board for many years, and later headed the School of Health and the History of Medicine Institute. Throughout his long career he was an outstanding leader of scientific medicine and medical education in America.[21]

William Osler, not yet forty years of age, arrived in Baltimore as Professor of Medicine in May, 1889. Dr. Henry M. Hurd became Superintendent of the Hospital in August 1889 at the age of forty-six. Hurd relieved the University President, Gilman, who had initially assumed the administration of the hospital. Osler nominated his young colleague from Philadelphia, Howard A. Kelly, who then was chosen to be Professor of Gynecology and Obstetrics at Johns Hopkins. He had an outstanding career as surgeon, teacher and writer.

William S. Halsted reached eminence as a surgeon and investigator at Bellevue Hospital. His successful demonstration of nerve block and spinal anesthesia with cocaine resulted in his own habituation to the drug. Welch aided his recuperation by encouraging him to work in the laboratories at Baltimore. Halsted was appointed Acting Surgeon of the Hospital in April, 1889 and Surgeon-in-Chief a year later. In 1892, Halstead who had promulgated important principles of surgery with wide applications, was promoted from Associate Professor to Professor of Surgery. He achieved fame through meticulous handling of tissues and innovative operating techniques, which he first perfected in the experimental surgical laboratory.[22]

While Halsted's full appointment was still pending, William Osler initiated the graded residency system in North America, which was modeled on what he had experienced in German medical centers. For the first year, Osler chose H.A. Lafleur from Montreal as Resident Physician and H. Toulmin and D.M. Reese from Philadelphia as assistant residents. Other hospital positions were soon filled, and the graded residency system was used in each service. Several of the early chief residents held the position for prolonged terms, but the usual training in medicine covered four or five years. Halsted, Kelly, and Osler each trained many successful pupils. Halsted selected several from his residents to develop the surgical subspecialties at Johns Hopkins; for example, Hugh Young in urology and Harvey Cushing in neurosurgery.

In the early days of the Johns Hopkins Hospital, Welch, Osler, Kelly and Halsted and the younger men worked together closely. Beginning in 1889, they shared ideas about the scientific and the humanistic aspects of medicine at weekly meetings of the Johns Hopkins Medical Society. The following year, meetings of the Historical Club were initiated by Osler with the regular participation of Welch, Billings, and Kelly. Men from other services, like Harvey Cushing, were strongly influenced by William Osler. His deep knowledge of the modern and past literature of medicine was freely shared to suggest further leads to every eager student and visiting practitioner. His pupils and other young associates soon named Osler "The Chief".

The Johns Hopkins Hospital Dispensary and Wards opened during the spring and summer of 1889, but the medical school did not commence instruction until September 1893. In September 1890, he began writing, and by ahering to an arduous schedule, he completed *The Principles and Practice of Medicine.* [23] in February, 1892. Though it consumed much of his time, Osler, repeatedly revised this successful textbook, and it earned him a considerable income throughout his life. This book was based on extensive personal experience. It immediately gained popularity with students and practitioners in America and abroad because of its organization and straightforward, but engaging, style. Osler was frank; the etiology of few of the major illnesses was understood, and highly effective specific medications were limited, quinine for malaria, digitalis for heart failure, mercury for syphilis, iron for anemia, opium for pain, and iodine for some types of goiter, for example. Some general practitioners accused Osler of being a therapeutic nihilist. On the other hand, Osler's book convinced Mr. F.T. Gates of the need for increased knowledge of the epidemic and other morbid afflictions of mankind. Gates initiated the proposal to John D. Rockefeller to begin his benefactions to medical research. Under the subsequent leadership of William Welch and other imaginative medical scientists, the Rockefeller Institute for Medical Research, and later, the Rockefeller Foundation, came into being.

After he had put the finishing touches on his textbook, and presented the first published copy to his friend from Philadelphia, William Osler slipped away from Baltimore for two weeks without revealing the purpose publicly. On May 7, 1892, Grace Linzee Revere Gross and William Osler were married without guests in St. James Church, Philadelphia. They spent their honeymoon meeting relatives and friends in New York, Boston, Toronto and Montreal. The deep affection which bound their married life is seen in their correspondence to the families and others, and is also referred to in Cushing's biography. Grace's father was descended from the American patriot, Paul Revere, and her mother from a British Navy Captain. As daughter-in-law of the famous Jefferson Medical College surgeon, Samuel D. Gross, and wife of his son and successor, Samuel W. Gross, she was accustomed to the role of companion and hostess for a medical professor with many friends and interests. An accomplished household manager and talented hostess, she adapted without known remonstrance to William Osler's habits of asking out of town professors to spend the nights at their home, bringing young students for the evenings to his library, and inviting large groups of professional acquaintances to tea or dinner.

Shortly after their hospitable meals, Osler withdrew to his office in the house. He entrusted all the details of these functions to his wife, who usually had arranged for daughters of friends or relatives to help her entertain the guests. Over the years, William and Grace Osler became devoted to several of these young women, treating them as daughters, and thus, sisters for their only son, Revere. Grace Osler took great satisfaction and pride in her husband's professional successes. She cheerfully agreed that young colleagues be given latchkeys to enter the house at No. 1 West Franklin Street in Baltimore, and their later homes, at their convenience for reading and consultation. She also developed mutually stimulating friendships with many of the latchkeyers and other young visitors.

While at times of crises, Osler suppressed his feelings with an outward calm, his devotion to his only son was always apparent, if casually expressed. Grace was moved by the deepest maternal love and concern, but as a wise and emotionally mature woman, she adjusted to the smaller problems, and even accepted the ultimate tragedy of their son's death, with less psychological and physical upset than did the father.

Though troubled in her later years by periods of arthralgia, perhaps due to gout, she remained strong physically until the late years of her widowhood. She suffered one premonitory stroke in December 23, 1927, and died of a massive hemiplegia on August 31, 1928, at the age of seventy-four years. Arnold Muirhead wrote an excellent biographical sketch, and George Harrell a delightful essay, "Lady Osler".[14,24]

William Osler enjoyed the company of children throughout his life. Frequently he played pranks and told fanciful tales in installments to the children of his cousin Marian Francis in Montreal. Later he corresponded, sent presents and visited his young relatives whenever professional duties permitted. Without affectation, he played and responded with imagination to all children at their levels, easily sharing in their joy and laughter. These leisurely moments were the source of mutual delight; Osler found the children refreshing and they welcomed the return of their "grown up" partner in frolic. This aspect of Osler's personality is especially illustrated in passages in the biography by Edith Gittings Reid, and also in Cushing's *Life.* [25]

After Revere was born, Osler delighted in every moment with him and joined in games with his childhood companions. Grace Osler liked English literature and customs, and readily agreed that Revere would have a British education. This desire was one factor in their mutual decision to move to Oxford when Revere was nine years old. ,

The father encouraged and participated with the youthful Revere in many pastimes, for example, fishing and hunting butterflies. He may have hoped that Revere would follow his own progress from nature studies to biological science. He called Revere "Isaac Walton" or "Ike", as well as "Tommy", and then introduced him to *The Compleat Angler.* This became a favorite book and led Revere eventually to the love of classical English literature. Osler took pride in Revere's participation in team games at his preparatory school in Oxford, and later in his successes in building cabinets and model boats. The father's interest grew from amusement to delight as Revere's artistic talents developed from youthful ink sketches to etchings of historic buildings and the design of his own book-plate. The recognition of these talents in Revere, likely inherited from his maternal ancestors, made William Osler predict that his son would become an architect or artist.

William Osler frequently mentioned to correspondents Revere's difficulties with Latin and Greek. Although the parental concern may have been excessive, Revere was granted leave from school at Winchester for private tutoring in the classics in preparation for University matriculation. Revere passed the entrance examinations on the second attempt in April, 1914. By this time he had developed a keen interest in English literature and book-collecting.

Revere was reserved, and somewhat shy, but he formed close

friendships with boys such as Raleigh Parkin and Bob Emmons who shared his interests in fishing or books. He was well-liked by his cousins and other young women who visited their home at Oxford to help as hostesses. Military service in World War I, when he was barely nineteen years old, however, was an over-riding factor in Revere's social development. The details of the Oslers' activities during the war, and Revere's death in battle in August 1917, will be presented later. Thomas Keys and George Harrell have written sensitive articles on Revere Osler's life.[26]

Osler's abilities as a bedside teacher have been mentioned, but his success as a practicing physician must also be acknowledged. From 1893, the consulting practice he had carried from Philadelphia to Baltimore grew rapidly at his office in the West Franklin Street home. The residents, and often visiting physicians, observed him on the public and private wards at the Johns Hopkins Hospital. Throughout his tenure, the children's medical wards were included in his service.

The adult and young patients recognized his deep human interest, intelligence and persistence in using every means to attend to their problems, and attempt to relieve their pains and discomfort. Doctor Osler was quickly trusted and loved. He listened carefully to each patient, but skillfully evaded and withdrew himself from the garrulous or gossiping man or woman after an appropriate but kindly word. Osler sometimes entered a child's sick room on all fours. Beginning with an amusing game, interspersed by quiet questions and appropriate clinical examinations, he would make an unexpected gift, deliver words of encouragement and disappear, leaving happy smiles on the faces of his young friends. His visits to children were not always hurried. Osler was effective as a diagnostician, morale builder, comforter and friend of the mature patient or the child and parent. These traits are clear in Cushing's *Life of Sir William Osler,* and are charmingly expressed in the words of Edith Gittings Reid:

"Only Dickens could have been one with him with children or in the wards of the poorhouse, sitting beside the downtrodden, the lowly and the suffering. Only Dickens could have measured comprehendingly the sweetness and tenderness of the great heart of a child in the brilliant man, making all his rich endowment merely a setting for his humanity."[27]

The fame of the Hopkins Institutions grew during the sixteen years of Osler's residence in Baltimore, 1889–1905. He was very busy in his professorial duties and in private consultation practice.

In addition to his participation in the Association of American Physicians, American Pediatrics Society and other clinical societies, he was active in professional and lay associations concerned with public health. These included tuberculosis congresses and other groups at the local, national and international levels. His interest in their work, and donations of rare books, stimulated many medical librarians. In addition, his interest, and accompanying encouragement, included nursing and other allied health professions.

Whether serving on the wards or in the clinical laboratory, Osler's pupils were stimulated to study and write. They made presentations at the Johns Hopkins Hospital and other medical societies, and their work was published in the journals. Osler's senior medical residents were Henri A. Lafleur (1889–1891), William S. Thayer (1891–1898), Thomas B. Futcher (1898–1901), Thomas McCrae (1901–1904) and Rufus I. Cole (1904–1906), all of whom became prominent physicians and teachers. Distinction was also achieved by many others who served as assistant residents and house officers on Osler's medical service, Thomas Boggs, Charles Camac, and Campbell Howard, among them.

The author's central purpose is to show the unusually powerful influence William Osler exerted on the pupils he trained throughout his long medical career. He had a strong effect on young men and women while he was at McGill, Pennsylvania, Johns Hopkins and Oxford. He also influenced many medical students, colleagues, and visiting practitioners at these locations and on his journeys to other medical institutions and professional gatherings. At Johns Hopkins, however, the medical residency provided the opportunity for "The Chief" to tutor neophytes in the art, skills, science and general humanities related to medicine. The longer the pupil remained on the service, the greater this influence was likely to be. Joseph Pratt and Charles Camac had relatively brief contact with Osler at Johns Hopkins, but continued the association for many years through their respective careers. Osler's importance to each of these pupils has been recorded.[28, 29]

Campbell Howard spent a longer period on Osler's medical service in Baltimore. As the son of Palmer Howard, Osler's clinical teacher in Montreal, he had long felt Osler's influence in a special way, and this close relationship lasted throughout their later professional and personal lives. The author believes that a detailed review of Osler's effect on this favored pupil may interest others whose early lives were closely touched by personal contacts or the teachings of William Osler, and also members of the later generations of medical professors and their pupils.

William Osler revered his own teachers and took pleasure in the injunction of Hippocrates to instruct the sons of his teachers and his colleagues. Of his three most honored teachers, James Bovell had daughters, but no son. The Reverend Mr. Johnson's elder son, Arthur Jukes Johnson, had already commenced his premedical education in Toronto when Osler entered the school at Weston. The second son, named James Bovell Johnson, studied medicine at McGill College where Osler assisted him with characteristic generosity. Immediately after graduating from McGill in 1876, he went to England where he shortly gave up the medical profession to enter the priesthood.[30]

Palmer Howard's older son, Jared, won Osler's prize of a microscope for excellence in his laboratory and clinical courses in 1881, and during the summer of 1884 they travelled and studied in Europe together. Osler undoubtedly played a part in Jared Howard's early professional development, but he concentrated his interests on surgery. Their professional careers thereafter were distinct, but the friendship between them and their families was renewed when the Oslers encountered them in 1905, living in England. Osler had the opportunity to train in internal medicine only one child of his three special teachers. The pupil was Campbell Howard.

Osler gave Campbell Howard opportunities in a gradual, thoughtful manner. He prodded, set tasks and encouraged in due measure. The road to the goal ahead required concentration and hard work, but central to the powerful relationship was the spirit of friendship and confidence between leader and follower, chief and pupil.

Campbell Howard worked hard in his medical courses and was graduated from the McGill College of Medicine in June, 1901. He interned at the Montreal General Hospital (M.G.H.) during the following year. On August 21, 1901, William Osler wrote him:

"I am delighted to think that you shall be in the old M.G.H. on Sept. 1st. How long is your service, 1 or 1-1/2 years? I think if you wish it I could arrange to take you on my service next year (after finishing at the M.G.H.). You would come in as one of the four senior Residents &

the work would be mainly bacteriological but you would see all the work & have to help in the teaching. If you think of it as likely, pay special attention to bacteriology this winter with [John] McCrae your Resident Pathologist —in fact it would be well to get him to coach you. Of course, if you think two years of Hospital work too much, with what you wish to spend abroad, it might be possible to arrange for some special work, but you would not have the advantage of living in the Hospital.

"Aunt Grace & Revere send love. We sail Sept. 14th."

John McCrae was then pathologist at the M.G.H., after previous study with William Osler and W.H. Welch in Baltimore. Campbell apparently accepted Osler's offer quite promptly. On September 27, Osler wrote again:

"I am writing [John] McCrae to keep an eye on you, and I know you will be able to pick up a good deal of practical knowledge. I think a year with us would probably be most useful. You would not be overworked, and could get out one or two good papers."

John McCrae probably approved the laboratory studies of a patient with quartan malaria, whose case history Campbell Howard reported during his internship in Montreal. On June, 1902, he began his training as assistant resident physician at Johns Hopkins Hospital with one year in the clinical laboratory (Figure 13). During that year W. S. Thayer and T. B. Futcher were Associates in Medicine, Thomas McCrae, resident physician, R. I. Cole and C.P. Emerson were the other assistant resident physicians, while twelve house officers covered the Hopkins Hospital services.

In the summer of 1903, Campbell Howard took his share of direct responsibilities on the wards and was appointed Assistant in Medicine on the Faculty. He replaced McCrae as instructor of the "Medical Anatomy" course. After October, 1904, T. McCrae was promoted to Associate in Medicine, Cole replaced him as Resident Physician, and T. R. Boggs was a new assistant resident physician. (31) The faculty and the young physicians in the Department of Medicine are shown in Figure 14.

Osler expressed his satisfaction with Campbell's progress in his July 13, 1904 letter. He was enjoying trout fishing with the eight-year-old Revere near Murray Bay about one hundred miles below the city of Quebec, when he wrote:

"You will be glad of a holiday. That was pretty tough work on Ward C. but wonderfully good for you in many ways. It is a great pleasure to have you with us & your future in Medicine should be assured. It would be better to go back to Montreal with a good reputation behind you in some good bits of clinical work accomplished."

At this time Osler also included the commendation, "Campbell H. is a great success. Working like a Trojan" in a letter to C. F. Martin, an influential professor of medicine at McGill.[32] Early in July, Osler also lunched with his former resident, H. A. Lafleur, who was then a Professor and senior physician at the Montreal General Hospital.[33] Good recommendations from "The Chief" assured Campbell's appointment to the medical staff of the "out-door" (outpatient) division of the Montreal General Hospital one year later. It was no longer necessary to confirm the appointment by canvassing all the contributors, or "governors" of the Hospital, a system which Osler accepted with reluctance when elected a hospital physician in 1878.[34] Campbell Howard acknowledged his appointment, but did not commence the duties until March, 1907.

A trans-Atlantic journey of great significance to William Osler and the medical world began light-heartedly on July 16, 1904. The *Campania* sailed from New York with several doctors. Thomas McCrae, Harvey Cushing, and Campbell Howard accompanied Osler. After long hours each day reading and writing papers in his cabin, Osler assembled the ship's surgeon, Francis Verdon, and all the medical friends aboard into the North Atlantic Medical Society. This met daily at tea-time for convivial discussion and banter. On the last evening of the trip, each member presented a nautical topic of dubious scientific character, invoking witty jibes. Osler later composed and distributed printed programs of the twelve presentations. These included, "The Minimal Lymph Pressure in the Ampullae as a Cause of Sea-sickness" by H. Cushing, "On Broadbent's Theory of Steady Dextral Cerulean Vision as a Preventative in the Disease" by William Osler, and "On the Chemistry of Aqua-Verdin; a New Gastro-Cutaneous Sea-Pigment" by Campbell Howard.[35]

Osler and his Baltimore colleagues visited London briefly before he presented a paper on pleurisy at the British Medical Association meeting in Oxford. Along with T. C. Allbutt, Patrick Manson and other prominent medical men, Osler was honored with the Doctor of Science degree from Oxford University. During the meeting, British medical leaders and Oxford University officials urged Osler to consider the Regius Professorship. The position was formally offered a few days later by Prime Minister Balfour. Mindful of Grace Osler's cable; "Do not procrastinate accept at once", he requested two weeks' delay before the announcement, and a year before he would take over the new duties at Oxford.[36]

Osler deeply regretted the prospect of leaving the stimulating colleagues and superb medical environment of the Johns Hopkins Institutions. Many friends knew that he felt severely strained from the increasing professional duties and consultations, but only his wife was aware that he was suffering symptoms of angina pectoris. He looked forward to a quieter life in Oxford and he also mentioned in a letter to his mother; "It will be much better for Revere . . .". To his colleague, W. S. Thayer, he remarked: "We can have a last good winter's work together, before I lapse into a quiet academic life."[37]

While his young companions returned promptly to their hospital work after the adventuresome journey, Osler spent several weeks with Grace, visiting their relatives and friends until later in September. His last academic year in Baltimore was fully occupied with clinical and teaching responsibilities, but he accepted requests for a large number of lectures, "farewell addresses" and presentations at the institutions and professional societies in which he had long played a leading role. Eighteen articles comprise the first edition of *Aequanimitas With Other Addresses,* published in October, 1904. For the second edition he added four addresses presented to his North American colleagues and students during 1905. The themes of most essays in this collection are timeless, and for many tomorrows these writings will convey Osler's inspiration to every reader from the medical and associated professions.

The lead article is from his Valedictory Address at the University of Pennsylvania in May, 1889. This contains advice for personal equanimity, or imperturbability, in all professional activities, not only to keep the trust of the patients, but to pass gently through the trials of life. "Doctor and Nurse" and "Nurse and Patient" were delivered in the 1890s at the Johns Hopkins Hospital. "Teacher and Student" was presented in 1892 at Minnesota, one

of the early tax-supported medical schools, and offers several comments still useful for State University Regents and administrators,
and many hints to help students everywhere. "Books and Men"
was delivered at the Boston Medical Library. It stresses the price-
less value of fine books to student, practitioner and teacher. "The
Leaven of Science", "Teaching and Thinking", "The Hospital as
a College", and "The Educational Value of the Medical Society"
each contain thought-provoking passages for educators and practitioners in various branches of our calling. The theme of "The
Master-Word in Medicine", delivered to medical students entering the University of Toronto in 1903, is surely still applicable
today to every scholar in the medical and health-related professions: aspiration can only be realized by diligent "work".

One of the four new essays, "The Fixed Period", delivered to
his friends at Johns Hopkins in February, 1905, was understood by
his audience, but misinterpreted by the public press. Osler's deep
regret about this prompted his explanatory remarks in the preface
to the 1906 edition of *Aequanimitas:*

> ". . . To relieve a situation of singular sadness in part-
> ing from my dear colleagues of the Johns Hopkins Univer-
> sity, I jokingly suggested for the relief of a senile profes-
> soriate an extension of Anthony Trollope's plan
> mentioned in his novel. . . ."

Throughout his youth and in his later life, Osler frequently demonstrated his devotion to older men. Here he extended his regrets
to any whose spirit he might have bruised. We may accept
the sincerity of his belief that he and other men usually do their
"real work of life" before forty years of age and should retire after
sixty.[38]

Each of the other three new essays included much wise advice
from the experienced professor. "The Student Life" was directed
to his former American and Canadian medical students. This was
first delivered at McGill University on April 14, 1905, and a little
later at the University of Pennsylvania. The memorable essay pro-
vides hints for the student aflame with the passion for knowledge.
To reach the truth requires an absorbing desire, an unswerving
pursuit and an open honest heart. For the student-practitioner, he
emphasized the need to study men as well as books, and he quoted
Cowper to distinguish between knowledge and wisdom. Much of
the advice and many of the models he held before the student-

specialist and the student-teacher are ideas which medical students, young and old, might reread with pleasure and profit.[39]

"Unity, Peace and Concord" was delivered in Maryland, but addressed to the medical profession of the United States. Osler pointed out the unity of interests and aims between all physicians; the ways to attain personal peace through overcoming ignorance, apathy and vice; and the nobleness of concord in a united profession by suppressing jealousy, or heeding detrimental tales about a brother physician. In summary, he offered each of his colleagues a single word—"charity".

The last chapter in *Aequanimitas* is "L'Envoi". This is based on brief remarks at a farewell dinner tendered him in New York by the medical profession of the United States and Canada on May 2, 1905. Filled with grateful recollections, Osler noted a few aspects of the profession in need of improvement, and then mentioned three personal ideals—to do the day's work well, to observe the Golden Rule towards professional brethren and patients, and "to cultivate such a measure of equanimity as would enable me to bear success with humility, the affection of my friends without pride and to be ready when the day of sorrow and grief came to meet it with the courage befitting a man."[40] From the deep sorrow of his last years, his friends would have yearned to spare him.

William Osler kept up with his heavy academic and professional activities during the fall and winter of 1904–05. A new edition of his textbook was also due. Friends, patients, colleagues and pupils needed advice and guidance from "The Chief". He regularly, and astutely, helped each young associate to study the clinical problems in the patients under their care. Thus, he undoubtedly stimulated and coordinated Campbell Howard's studies and reports on three patients with pneumococcic arthritis in 1903, and on peptic ulcers in 1904–05. He suggested that Campbell's paper, "The Incidence of Gastric Ulcer in America", be on the program of the June, 1904 meeting of the American Gastro-Enterological Association. The more significant clinical study of 82 cases of peptic ulcer was published later in 1904 from Osler's clinic. During the winter of 1905, Campbell read a paper at the Philadelphia County Medical Society and two before the Johns Hopkins Medical Society. After the last paper, when he reviewed seven case reports and presented the history of a patient with gastric tetany, W. G. MacCallum described the pathological lesion and described the differential diagnosis.[41] Osler had Campbell's experience in mind on March 23, 1905, when he wrote:

"I wish you would look over the section on the stomach in my text-book, particularly the chronic gastritis and the neuroses, and see if you could not suggest and add something. The sooner the better."

This was dictated while Osler was recovering from a week in bed with influenza and bronchitis. After additional time convalescing in Atlantic City, he returned to write a congratulatory note to his newly appointed successor, Lewellys F. Barker, who had been an assistant resident physician in 1891–92, and who had long served in the Johns Hopkins Hospital's pathology department before his illustrious years in basic science at the University of Chicago. Osler mentioned the increasing load of teaching, ward and private clinical work at the hospital, and described the attributes and responsibilities of each of the senior associates and resident physicians.[42]

Campbell Howard soon completed Osler's assignment for the textbook. Several parts of the section on the stomach in the book were revised in line with Campbell's articles. In the preface to the 6th edition of *The Principles and Practice of Medicine* dated May 17, 1905, Osler included Campbell Howard on the list of those who helped him. He acknowledged the special assistance of T. B. Futcher, T. McCrae and C. P. Emerson and singled out H. M. Thomas and Harvey Cushing for their contributions on the nervous system. Osler gave Campbell the autographed "Presentation Copy", number 19 (Figure 16).

PREFACE TO SIXTH EDITION.

So many sections have been rewritten, and so many alterations made, that in many respects this is a new book. The publishers have furnished a larger page and new type, so that with a considerable increase in the amount of reading matter there has been no enlargement of the volume. I have tried to make the work a reflex of current knowledge in the symptomatology and treatment of disease, based upon the literature and upon our experience at the Medical Clinic of the Johns Hopkins Hospital. During the sixteen years of its existence I have been singularly fortunate in my associates and assistants whose good work has been incorporated in the various editions. It would be useless to attempt to express my indebtedness to them—to H. M. Thomas, Henri Lafleur, W. S. Thayer, John Hewetson, Meredith Reese, Charles E. Simon, T. B. Futcher, Frank R. Smith, T. McCrae, C. P. Emerson, C. N. B. Camac, Rufus I. Cole, T. R. Brown, Louis P. Hamburger, Campbell P. Howard, T. R. Boggs, J. Erlanger, and others whose names will be found scattered through the volume. In this edition I am under special obligations to T. B. Futcher, T. McCrae, C. P. Emerson, and more particularly to H. M. Thomas, of the Neurological Department, and to Harvey Cushing, of the Surgical Clinic, who have revised the section on the Nervous System.

Upon my colleagues in other departments of the hospital I have drawn freely for advice. I am much indebted to Dr. W. H. Welch and to W. G. McCallum and to MacLeod Harris (now of Chicago).

I have to thank my fellow teachers in the medical schools of the English-speaking world for the warm reception which they have accorded to the previous editions. But, above all, I appreciate most highly the encouragement and support of the general practitioners throughout the country with whom the work has brought me into such close contact. I have to thank my nephew, W. W. Francis, for reading the proofs. To my secretary, Miss B. O. Humpton, who has again prepared the index, I am deeply indebted for an unceasing interest in the work ever since, in 1890–91, I dictated to her the first edition.

WILLIAM OSLER.

JOHNS HOPKINS HOSPITAL, *May 17, 1905.*

THE FAMILY OF ROBERT PALMER HOWARD, M.D.

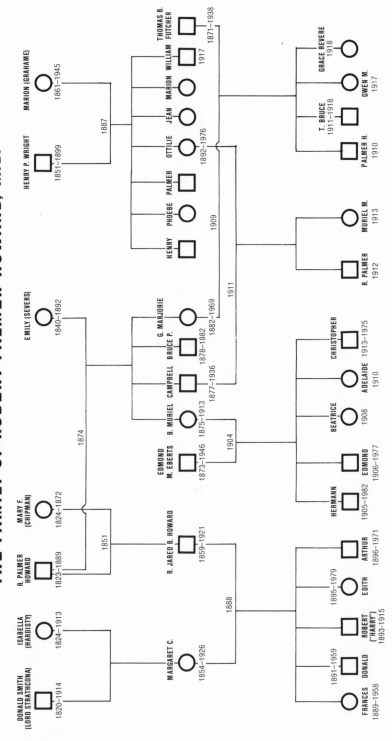

CHAPTER III

Regius Professor
of Medicine, Oxford

OSLER'S LAST WEEKS in America were overcrowded with professional obligations and farewells. As indicated by a note to Campbell Howard on May 8 about photographs and information concerning patients with abdominal tumors, he was already looking ahead to his professional commitments in Britain. He left to his efficient wife all the details concerned with leaving their home in Baltimore and moving to Oxford. Osler completed the revisions for the sixth edition of his textbook a few days before he went to Washington for meetings of two important medical societies. He had been a leading figure in them since their founding, and that year his friend, E. L. Trudeau, was serving as the President of both societies. The Association of American Physicians and the newer National Association for the Study and Prevention of Tuberculosis met from May 16 through May 18. Osler contributed to the scientific discussions, gave an address, and was bade farewell by his devoted fellow physicians. William Osler sailed the next day on the *Cedric* with his wife, Grace, Revere, Marjorie Howard, Arnold Klebs, Thomas McCrae and W.S. Thayer. The Oslers began their Oxford sojourn May 27, 1905, in a spacious furnished house at 7 Norham Gardens owned by the widow of Professor F. Max Müller.[43]

The letters from William Osler at Oxford to Campbell Howard further reveal the special relationship between "The Chief" and his pupil. Together with those to Marjorie Howard, the letters also shed much light on William Osler's professional and family activities. First, however, I will present a brief overview of Osler's responsibilities as the Regius Professor in Oxford University, and of his many professional activities from his arrival to the onset of World War I. These details may be found in Cushing's biography.

After a few days of rest, Osler began to participate in the academic and medical activities of Oxford. In contrast to the hustle and bustle of an American city, Oxford, at that time, was a venerable country town of 50,000 inhabitants. Life centered on a scattered group of Colleges, many of whose traditions emanated from the 16th century. While the Oslers loved the traditions they encountered, the Oxford dons and scholars soon discovered that the new Regius Professor of Medicine brought a vitality which always invigorated and sometimes subtly altered the time-honored activities. William Osler's influence spread in a short time from the Oxford nidus throughout the United Kingdom.

He was delighted to become a "Student" of Christ Church, a College renowned for its illustrious members. He was also elected to the Hebdomadal Council, which deliberated and initiated legislation for the University, serving faithfully for the first three years he was at Oxford. W. Osler devoted much of his talent and energy to Bodley's Library as a Curator, not only by raising contributions, but supporting the daily activities and stimulating the library staff. He also served gladly as a delegate to the Clarendon Press. Grace Osler shared his pleasure in the responsibilities of the Regius as Master of the ancient Alms-house at Ewelme.

William Osler enthusiastically encouraged many activities at the Radcliffe Library and the Infirmary. As Regius Professor, he presided at the hospital staff meetings and frequently visited the wards and laboratories. He brought experienced leadership, marked by his delightful tact and wit, to all areas of the Infirmary. Practitioners from the town and countryside flocked to join the scholarly medical rounds each week, and all recognized Osler's clinical acumen and personal interest in his colleagues. He accepted calls for consultations and led the organization of branch meetings of the British Medical Association and other health groups, notably the Oxfordshire branch of the National Association for the Prevention of Consumption.[44]

The Regius was Chairman of the Board of the Faculty of Medicine at Oxford University and responsible for the examination of the undergraduates. Osler participated in expanding and modernizing the facilities and teaching capabilities of the laboratory sciences, such as pharmacology and pathology. Courses in clinical subjects were not formally offered to undergraduates at Oxford during Osler's period. However, he instructed small groups of students weekly on the elements of the patient history and physical examination. He also invited them to his home where he illustrated important aspects of medicine from his modern and ancient classical books.

Early in 1907, the Oslers occupied thier own home at 13 Norham Gardens. The house was extensively renovated to include a consultation office, a library, sleeping accomodations for several guests, and adequate space for entertaining. Usually the weather allowed guests to spread over the terrace and large lawn. William Osler and his gracious wife entertained so often that their home was called "The Open Arms". Rhodes Scholars from United States, Canada and elsewhere shared in this hospitality, and received an introduction to English life and advice on their own academic interests.

Osler gladly contributed helpful suggestions for the scientific investigations of his colleagues or younger students, and arranged for collaborative studies on the wards and laboratories of the Radcliffe Infirmary. Osler's influence at Oxford is illustrated by his continued participation in the pathology laboratory with A. G. Gibson, and in the history of science room at the Radcliffe Library with Charles Singer. Osler inspired many other young men and women in Oxford, as previously, to forge ahead to a specific set of professional and personal goals, their path in life.[45]

By tradition, Regius Professors of Medicine at Oxford and Cambridge were leading representatives of the profession throughout the United Kingdom. Osler frequently visited Cambridge and felt a deep respect and affection for his "Brother Regius", Sir T. Clifford Allbutt, whose tribute to Osler revealed reciprocal sentiments.[46] Osler was a Fellow of the Royal Society. He was also often in London as a Fellow of the Royal College of Physicians, or visiting physician at one of the city hospitals. He contributed notable lectures on topics of disease, public health, education or professional organization. His Harveian Oration at the Royal College of Physicians on October 18, 1906, is a conspicuous example among his many eminent addresses.

Osler also participated in the organization of the Royal Society of Medicine, and he served as president of the Clinical Section as well as the founder and first president of the History of Medicine section. He frequently participated in international meetings throughout his career, and he served as President of the Medical Section at the International Medical Congress in London in 1913. Osler also enjoyed the companionship of men in many vocations at the Athenaeum and other clubs in London and Oxford.

He was an active participant and often a leading speaker at the British Medical Association's annual meetings which were held in many different cities. He also lectured at medical schools in Manchester, Edinburgh, Dublin and elsewhere. He played a major part in the organization of the Association of Physicians of Great Britain and Ireland in 1907. His energy and tact also contributed to the founding of a publication in the special field of internal medicine, *The Quarterly Journal of Medicine.* Osler remained one of the journal's six editors throughout his life. He also helped found a British association of medical librarians.

In the ancient college environment of Oxford, Osler used his leisure to supplement and arrange his library in a manner to illustrate the significant events in medical history. He bequeathed this Bibliotheca Osleriana to McGill University where it eventually became the nidus of the Osler Library at his alma mater. After his extensive involvement with the hectic medical environment in America, the Oxford move appeared eminently satisfactory and beneficial to his health. His account book reveals, however, that he missed "the active teaching & the close association with students and a large group of young doctors, but I console myself with the 31 years of strenuous work I had in Canada & the United States."(47)

Close to his humanistic and literary interests were the meetings of the Bibliographical Society and the Classical Association. Remarkably, as a physician, he was elected President of each, and served with conspicuous success. In 1914, he read the presidential address, "Incunabula Medica; a Study of the Earliest Printed Medical Books (1467–1480)" and it was published posthumously by the Bibliographical Society with extensive notes by V. Scholderer of the British Museum. Osler's address to the Classical Association will be discussed later.

Osler had studied in Berlin and Vienna in 1873–74 and maintained his ties with German medicine thereafter. His location in Oxford allowed frequent meetings with leading German and Austrian clinicians such as F. von Müller, C. A. Ewald, F. Kraus, L. Krehl, and K. F. Wenckebach. Osler formed friendships with these men which even the Great War would not break.

From his arrival in Oxford until World War I, it was important

to Osler that he maintain his ties at home, and he made time for
trips to the United States and Canada. Most of his own family
resided in Toronto, or elsewhere in Canada, and his wife's relatives lived near Boston. Deep ties of personal and professional
friendship drew him to his former Universities in Toronto, Montreal, Philadelphia, and Baltimore. These transoceanic trips in 1905,
1906, 1907, 1909, 1910 and 1913 contained few unscheduled hours.
Keeping abreast of the progress in American medical education,
and of the careers of former colleagues, assistants and younger
members in the health-related fields stimulated his professional
acumen and rekindled his inspirational influence on this side of
the Atlantic.

Conspicuous events from his last trip to America illustrate the
remarkably wide range of his interests and contributions. On April
15–17, 1913, Osler shared in the opening of the Phipps Psychiatric
Clinic at Johns Hopkins Hospital, where he spoke on "Specialism
in the General Hospital". Later he returned to Baltimore to talk
at the Nursing School Commencement. Between these events he
delivered the inspirational message, "A Way of Life", to Yale students on April 20. During the week he lectured there for the
Silliman Foundation, except for one day at the memorial meeting
for John S. Billings in New York. Publication of the Silliman Lectures was delayed by the war but effected by his friends in 1921
under the title, *The Evolution of Modern Medicine.* [48]

The first letter Campbell Howard received from Oxford, dated
June 2, 1905, began:

> "We arrived safely on Saturday night [May 27] and
> found a very comfortable house with good servants. It
> was awfully dull the first two days and quiet, so that
> Tommy [Revere] had a constant desire to scream. We are
> now getting into pretty good shape, but it will take
> months to settle down. . . ."

Osler then referred again to the necessary collaboration of his
former Johns Hopkins associates in preparing his next lecture. H.
M. Little was in J. W. Williams' department of obstetrics and J. C.
Bloodgood in surgery. W. O. wrote:

> "You did find out the figures of the abdominal tumors,
> did you not? I would like copies of them all. I am prepar-
> ing a lecture on the subject, and have an article for Keen's

New System of Surgery. I wish you would ask "Butch" [H.M. Little] to look over the figures in their department and let me have anything that is specially striking or useful. Ask [J.C.] Bloodgood if you could not look over his list. There were two cases of huge sarcoma of the abdomen from retained orchids [testicles]."

Osler mentioned the photographs and reports of abdominal tumors in cryptorchid patients in his August 13, August 24 and December 13, 1905 letters to Campbell. On the reverse of the August 13 letter are hospital chart and surgical pathology numbers in Campbell Howard's handwriting. These referred to the two subjects whose case reports illustrated Osler's lecture at the Radcliffe Infirmary on March 20, 1907, and which were presumably included in the unpublished Thomas Young Lectures at Saint George's Hospital in London during June 1906.[49]

In his July 22, 1905 letter Osler made a request for assistance in another topic, and later he thanked Campbell:

"I wish you would send me the photograph of William Smith, the aneurysm of the abdominal aorta. I think there were a couple taken, one, also, towards the end when he had the leg drawn up. . . ."
"All right about Smith's photo—twill do quite well."

The article on aneurysm was published.[50]

Osler had also mentioned that he was busy with the examinations of the medical students in Oxford. For this first experience of the new Regius his friends, G.A. Gibson of Edinburgh and G. Schorstein of the London Hospital, examined in medicine. He also reported frequent visits to London. An important reason was sitting for the famous portrait by John S. Sargent, which Miss Mary Garrett commissioned for the Johns Hopkins Hospital. He remarked that he had "a somewhat saturnine face", but he was more pleased with this than the original one painted by Thomas Cromwell Corner (he later improved it) for the Medical and Chirurgical Faculty of Maryland.[51]

Though busy in and out of Oxford through July, the three Oslers spent August 15–September 8, 1905, in the Highlands of Scotland. Each of them enjoyed the hospitality and scenery, while Revere was happiest fishing with his father on the mountain streams. Near their old friend Henry Phipps' Beaufort Castle, W.

O. wrote Campbell that "Ike caught some trout & landed a huge pike about which he dreams & talks all the time." The Oslers also spent a week on the Island of Colonsay, which Lord Strathcona had recently acquired. The spacious manor house was often used by his daughter, wife of Palmer Howard's elder son, Jared, and Marjorie Howard was visiting the family at that time.

After returning to Oxford, Osler was soon busy with professional activities. His election as "Student", or Fellow, at Christ Church brought him rooms for his personal use. Grace and William Osler took great pleasure in furnishing them, as the letter by three writers to Campbell on Sunday, October 29, 1905, confirms:

> [from Grace Osler] "Docci O's new old desk is being used for the first time to send a line to you. Marjorie is with us. We have just come from the Service in the Cathedral & Reggie [W.Osler] has gone into his own stall arrayed in surplice & hood and winking at M & me as he came down the aisle. I wish you could see the rooms—they are really charming and it has been great fun getting them in order. We are now looking forward to showing you all the treasures of Oxford and particularly your godson [Revere]— who is rapidly becoming an English boy with an accent."
> [from Marjorie Howard] "Oh! such fun! You really have never seen anyone as killing as our Reggie! I'm so happy to be back here, & if you were only here too, it would be perfect. Reggie has just danced a shirt dance in his surplice."
> [from William Osler] "These old fools have put me in a surplice & I had to go to chapel, but I wished I had been in the pulpit instead of the Regius Prof. of Divinity who is a dry old stick."

From Marjorie Howard's later recollections, she was the first to coin the flippant nickname "Reggie" from the impressive title, Regius Professor. Thereafter, Osler frequently signed "Reggie" in letters to Marjorie. The "new old desk" was later moved into Revere's room at 13 Norham Gardens. By Grace Osler's will, it was left to T. Archibald Malloch, whose descendants recently donated it to the Osler Library at McGill University.[52]

We now leave William Osler and his family as they adjusted so successfully to their new life in Oxford and return to his interest in Campbell Howard's progress. From their discussions in Baltimore, Osler was aware that Campbell planned a year's study in Europe after he had arranged to end his activities as assistant resident in medicine at Johns Hopkins. The Oslers had planned to spend several weeks in December and January visiting kinfolk and professional colleagues in America. Osler wrote to Campbell on August 3, 1905:

> "Let me know what you have settled about your plans. I shall be in Baltimore for the month of January. It would be nice if you and I came over together, if you did not intend to stay the winter. I think if you could have a few months with Müller in Munich, you could get out a good piece of work. I hope you will go over the question of dilated stomach. I am sure there is material enough for a very good article."

Friedrich von Müller had trained under famous contributors to metabolic research and internal medicine at Munich, Würzburg and Berlin. After establishing himself as an outstanding teacher of the scientific approach to internal medicine at several centers in Germany, he transferred in 1902 to Munich where his work established the fame of the II Medical Clinic. Campbell promptly decided to accept Osler's assistance in arranging for him to work with Müller, and joined him in Munich in March, 1906. Osler replied that he would request L. F. Barker, his Hopkins successor, to permit Campbell to terminate his position at the end of January.

In the letter of August 24, 1905, Osler also congratulated Campbell on the acceptance for publication by F.R. Packard of another article related to gastroenterology.[53] Campbell noted that six of the seven adult patients with tetany had evidence of gastric dilation, the other had chronic diarrhea, and the two children had rickets. His discussion included other causes of tetany and the benefit of parathyroid extract. Osler still encouraged Campbell to investigate further the relationship between the tetany and gastric dilation, but his investigations in Munich, and later, were on other subjects.

Campbell may not have requested, but certainly welcomed, his mentor's guidance in reporting cases of parotitis. In a postcard dated October 21, 1905, Osler referred to an article in the current issue of *Lancet.* He mentioned a patient of W.S. Halsted's and added: "The association of other glands as in Mikulicz disease should be referred to." Campbell later published a long review on the subject, including four new patients. One had consulted Osler in 1900, and the others entered Johns Hopkins Hospital between January and April, 1905, when Campbell was an assistant resident on Osler's service. He referred to a report by Osler in 1898, but did not specify any as W. S. Halsted's patients.[54]

The three Oslers sailed from Britain in time to join Grace's mother and family in Canton, Massachusetts on Christmas eve. His wife and Revere visited relatives until his schooling required them to sail home in the middle of January. Osler, however, went on to visit Maude Abbott at the McGill Medical Museum and his own mother and family in Toronto. For most of January, Osler was in Baltimore, but he also visited Philadelphia and New York. In Washington he attended a testimonial dinner for Robert Fletcher, compiler of *Index Medicus*. During his last weeks in Baltimore, he lived in the hospital where he made bedside clinical rounds, visited colleagues and participated in all groups of interest to him. He spent many hours with Thomas McCrae on assembling the contributions submitted for their *System of Medicine,* but probably found the greatest satisfaction in encountering the first patient in his experience with a variant of telangiectasia.

After this busy sojourn, he thanked his obliging hosts, including L.F. Barker, and sailed from New York on *The Campania* with Campbell Howard on February 3, 1906. His exhaustion contributed to a recurrence of respiratory infection.[55] However, he light-heartedly confided in a note to Marjorie Howard on March 16: ". . . . I have been back for a month, not in fine feather, a cold which I catched on the boat hung on for a couple of weeks & I dined one night in an ice-box and it came back." W. O. busied himself with letters and kept an engagement with the British Medical Association in London on February 16, where he lunched with his young protégé. Campbell had spent a few days in Oxford, visited his brother Jared in London, and then left England to start work with Müller in Munich.

For about five weeks, Campbell Howard settled in at Müller's Clinic in Munich. It was a wholly new environment for him, different in national, cultural, and professional terms. It is likely that he was so busy learning a new language, and so enthralled by the sights, sounds and customs of the old world city, that he had neglected writing to his godfather and "Chief". Osler began his letter to Campbell on April 3 in a parental manner: "How are you— where are you—what are you doing—where have you been—why don't you give an account of yourself?" He continued that the young Oxford practitioner, A. G. Gibson, would accompany him to Germany. Osler intended to help him improve his knowledge of pathology. They scheduled two days' stay in Marburg to study in Ludwig Aschoff's laboratory, especially the heart preparations. They also stopped at Frankfort to see Paul Ehrlich's laboratory. Osler must have considered that it was essential for a beginner in the specialty of pathology to learn to read the German literature for he requested Campbell to procure a small German manual of anatomy. The visitors arrived in Munich the evening before the German Congress for Internal Medicine opened in Munich on April 23, 1906. Osler attended the four-day meeting with his young colleagues and introduced them to prominent German physicians. Müller, of course, participated, and so did the Berlin professors with whom Campbell would later study, Carl Anton Ewald of gastric test meal fame, and Friedrich Kraus.[56]

W.O.'s brief notes in the next few months to Campbell in Munich included three requests. The first was to identify a German text with hematological plates for clinical diagnosis—Campbell named Emil Ponfick's *Topographischer Atlas . . .* , Jena, 1901. The second was to call on Smith Ely Jelliffe of New York, the contributor of chapters on migraine and hysteria to Osler and McCrae's *System of Medicine,* who was visiting Emil Kraeplin's Psychiatric Clinic in Munich. The third was to submit by November 1, 1906 a suitable contribution on arthritis to a series on their experience with pneumonia. For this Joseph A. Chatard (M.D., Johns Hopkins, 1903) assumed the responsibility. Campbell met the requested deadline, but the publication of the "fasciculus" by the associated contributors was delayed for several years.[57]

Campbell Howard spent over seven months with Müller in Munich. He completed a creditable piece of laboratory investigation under the guidance of Dr. Karl Stauvli on the eosinophilic cells. He read a short version before the Laboratory Section of the Canadian Medical Association in Montreal, September 13, 1907. In the full paper, he presented the response of the eosinophilic cells in the blood and tissues to a variety of salts, proteins, and toxic substances. W. O. wrote in January, 1908 to Campbell in Montreal: "I am greatly pleased with your paper in the Journal of Medical Research. It was a first rate piece of work and will increase your rising stock in the medical market."[58]

No letters from Osler to Campbell Howard are extant for July through September, 1906. He had mentioned that Marjorie Howard had returned to England and that the Oslers had to leave 7

Norham Gardens for Mrs. Max Müller to use in July. For part of the month, the Oslers stayed in The Master's rooms at Ewelme. They discovered in the safe, original documents of the 14th to 16th centuries, to the Master's great enjoyment. With the immediate aid of W.W. Francis and professional assistance at the Bodleian, the "Ewelme Muniments" were restored for permanent display. The Oslers obtained possession of their own house at 13 Norham Gardens on August 1, but many details concerned with its restoration and modernization of the plumbing, etc. occupied much of Osler's time and forced cancellation of other plans which included his attendance at the British Medical Association meeting in Toronto.[59]

Marjorie Howard joined her brother in Berlin in October, while Osler was "in the toils of that horrid address". The Harveian Oration, "The Growth of Truth as Illustrated in The Discovery of the Circulation of the Blood", was delivered on October 18, 1906, at the Royal College of Physicians in London. At the conclusion of his eloquent tribute to the life and work of the most famous Fellow of the College, Osler congratulated a contemporary. His friend and surgeon, Mr. Jonathan Hutchinson, was awarded the Moxon Medal of the College of Physicians at Osler's instigation. The Oration was followed by a ceremonial dinner to which Osler was allowed only two guests, Mr. Henry Phipps of New York and Lord Strathcona and Mount Royal, whom he had first met while at McGill University. Both men had continued their generous contributions to Osler's medical interests in Great Britain. In his October 19 letter to Marjorie Howard, Osler remarked about the Oration:

> "It seems to have been a great success—so they all said. I sent a card to R.J.B. [Howard] but I did not see him in the crowd. Strathie [Lord Strathcona] was at the dinner and most gracious. . . . I have Campbell's letter & will answer it tomorrow. I have not had a moment. I will send him a Lancet with the Oration. The Times gave it a column—most kind of them."[60]

Marjorie and Campbell Howard were introduced in Berlin by Osler's letter to the U.S. Embassy Secretary John Garrett, one of the Baltimore family so important to him and the Johns Hopkins medical institutions. He also wrote his physician friends, Ewald and Kraus. The three Oslers spent the holidays from December 6 through January 8, 1907 in America. W.O.'s itinerary included Baltimore, Hamilton, Ont., Toronto, Montreal, Boston for Christmas with the Reveres, Philadelphia, Baltimore again and New York. Suffice it here to mention that in Toronto the University officials offered him the presidency, which he politely refused. In Baltimore he gave an interesting address on the associations of the Warrington Collection, a part of which had been purchased by W. A. Marburg for the Johns Hopkins Medical School, and to which he had personally added a copy of the first edition (1628) of Harvey, *De motu cordis.* In New York, he joined in tributes given in memory of Dr. Mary Putnam Jacobi, an excellent pediatrician in her own right, and wife of his friend, Abraham. Osler remembered many other friends, old and young, during this journey as shown by the following letter to Marjorie Howard, which was written in January, 1907, about a week after their return to Oxford. Grace and William Osler lived for a short time in the King's Arms Hotel, and then they moved into 13 Norham Gardens, before the furnace and other utilities were in running order.[61]

"I had such a happy visit in Montreal. . . . All old friends seemed glad to see me. I put several spokes in Campbell's wheels with the senior men. He will be most heartily welcomed, and when he settles down will like it so much. There is a great future for the school & I know of no place with so many nice young fellows. The M G H is booming & C. will be so pleased with the Laboratories. . . . On my return visit [to Baltimore] I stayed with the [H.B.] Jacobs whose new house is enchanting. But wait until you see no. 13! & the vista from your room. You must stay as long as you possibly can. We should get in next week. Scottie & Tom [Revere] are there, camping out with the servants. My consulting room is ready but the workmen are still in the other parts. We had such a fine voyage—Kaizer W. [Wilhelm] der II—5d. & 11 hours to Plymouth. Term has not begun so the town is very dull. Did I tell C. that I have 1st Edition of Laennec for a Xmas present & not to forget it. I am sure he will have a profitable stay in Wien. Ask him to call on the Tetany man— what is his name [Anton von Eiselberg]. And would he like a letter to [C.] von Noorden or to [E. von] Neusser?

All my old friends are gone. We have not seen any of the
boys—but on Sunday they will be at the new house—the
Open Arms or the Always *Inn. . . .*"

Either of the suggested names for the Oslers' home would have
been appropirate. Possibly Marjorie and the Oslers had already
bandied these in conversation during Marjorie's recent visit to
Oxford. Much later Archibald Malloch expressed the view that the
designation "The Open Arms" was first given to the house by an
undergraduate. The name was habitually used from sometime in
1907 throughout the Oslers' occupancy.[62]

While in Vienna during January, 1907, Campbell visited the
hospitals and surely endeavored to see the work of Osler's acquaintances. He and Marjorie then went to Paris. Osler had sent
him letters of introduction to the world-famous Pierre Marie, who
described acromegaly, and other prominent physicians, Fulgence
Raymond, André Chantemesse and Octave Crouzon.

Marjorie and Campbell spent a few days enjoying the house
and lawns of "The Open Arms" and bidding farewell to the beloved Oslers. On February 22, 1907, Osler inscribed the fine
volumes by R.T.H. Laënnec, *De l'Auscultation Médiate* (Paris,
1819), "Campbell Howard, from Wm. Osler, Oxford", which are
now in the author's personal library. Campbell Howard had completed the formal stages of his professional education, and with his
sister, he sailed for Montreal to take up his appointment at the
Montreal General Hospital and in the medical laboratory under
the supervision of the McGill College of Medicine.

The McGill medical faculty at this time was composed of experienced leaders and a number of younger persons who sought
to institute more of the basic and clinical research methods of
contemporary medical schools. Osler had commented on this
spirit in his letters to Campbell Howard. Principal Peterson and
Osler frequently exchanged views on medical education.

At a faculty meeting late in 1906, changes were proposed to
reduce the number of didactic lectures in clinical subjects and to
add instruction in minor surgery and physicial diagnosis. These
suggestions were accepted by a committee composed of the Dean
and full professors of the departments of medicine, surgery, obstetrics and gynecology. The committee, however, rejected the
provision that, for each of these clinical departments, there should
be a salaried head who would pursue research work and teaching
and be permitted a consulting practice only. Principal Peterson

sent the Committee report to Osler with the implication that the opposition of many senior faculty was based on their consideration of the University's financial constraints rather than ideals of teaching. Osler's reply appears to favor all the initial recommendations:

> "I am sure the teaching in both medicine and surgery can be organized in this way, and it would be a great deal more satisfactory to the students. The other suggestions dealing with the didactic lectures, I approve of most heartily. Would it not be better to give the didactic lectures to the third year students and to arrange the work so that the fourth year students could be in the hospitals all day?"

However, the McGill Medical College did not institute a system of salaried heads for the clinical department for many years.[63]

Campbell and Marjorie Howard arrived in Montreal about the first of March, 1907. He soon bought a residence with office rooms on Mackay Street near St. Catherine Street. The location was nearly three miles from the Montreal General Hospital, but within a half-mile of McGill College and other doctors' offices. From the outset, he restricted his practice to medical consultations which few young practitioners since Osler had attempted in Montreal. Campbell did not have many referrals during the next three years, but busied himself with his out-patient duties, teaching and the establishment of a clinical chemistry laboratory at the College. There he performed investigative studies on patients in collaboration with the General Hospital's senior attending physicians, F. G. Finley and H. A. Lafleur.

Osler's letters to Campbell's sisters in Montreal frequently included praise and encouraging messages for him. On March 21, 1907, he deputized Muriel Eberts to purchase desks for both Campbell and Marjorie. He included the comment: "I am sure C. will be very happy when he gets into good steady work. He has had a splendid training and has such good judgment in matters medical that he will soon be found out."

In April, the McGill community and its supporters were shocked by a serious fire at the medical building. Dean Roddick immediately cabled McGill's Chancellor Lord Strathcona in London and Principal Peterson wrote him detailed information. Campbell also cabled Osler whose optimistic acknowledgement confirmed his imperturbability: "My only regret is about the books and specimens, though I hope a good many of them have been saved. In the long run it will be a very good thing. The old building was a compromise and too much patchwork about it." The medical building had been extended in 1893 through funds provided by Lord Strathcona, but most of the building was now destroyed, including portions of the medical museum and library. The building had to be rebuilt, and the $350,000 insurance covered only part of the loss. When Osler visited Montreal later in April, he found that many of his own specimens in the museum had survived. He saw the Howards and many of his friends in senior positions at McGill. From the first, Osler solicited endowments to support medical research in the proposed new facilities.[64]

In view of the warm friendship between Osler and Lord Strathcona, and the many other occasions when Osler's appeals were answered, it is probable that he explained his broad view of McGill's needs personally to Strathcona in support of the Principal's letters. Repairs were soon made on the surviving part of the old medical building. Construction of the new Strathcona medical building was completed during 1910 near the Royal Victoria Hospital at a cost approximating $600,000. After spending the insurance, the Chancellor's generous bequest of $450,000 allowed about $100,000 surplus. McGill University also received large gifts from Sir William Macdonald for other Colleges, but wider support was needed. At the Principal's request Osler agreed to solicit funds from other civic leaders, such as Henry Birks, and his patient James Ross, who had previously provided the money to build the private pavillon of the Royal Victoria Hospital.[65]

As soon as Osler reached Oxford after his North American trip he sent a characteristic postcard to Campbell with affectionate greetings from all the Oslers. Professor Julius Dreschfeld of Manchester had raised a question about acute myxedema. Osler suggested that Campbell send him a copy of his recent article in Volume 48 of the *Journal of the American Medical Association*, and in his next letter to Campbell he mentioned the professor's interest.

Campbell had been busily engaged in starting his outpatient duties at the Montreal General Hospital, and setting up a laboratory for clinical research, but he also undoubtedly participated actively in welcoming his Munich preceptor. Professor Friedrich von Müller visited Montreal twice during his tour of North American medical centers. While the guest of McGill's Dean T. G. Roddick in April, he gave a clinic on blood diseases and lectured on disseminated sclerosis at the Royal Victoria Hospital. The next day he spoke on pneumonia at the Montreal General Hospital. In the evening the guest compared German and American University methods of instruction. Müller returned for the award of the LL.D. degree honoris causa at the McGill University Convocation on June 12, 1907.[66] In Osler's October, 1907, letter to Campbell he enclosed a recent letter from Müller, and mentioned his gift of William Macmichael's *Gold-Headed Cane* to his fellow professor and friend.

During the summer of 1907, Osler attended the British Medical Association meeting in Exeter. He discussed papers by A. G. Robb on cerebrospinal fever and by J.S.R. Russell on the indications for operation on intracranial tumors; he also presented one on acute pancreatitis.[67] Osler mentioned the visits of T. McCrae, H. M. Hurd, Futcher and Boggs of Baltimore and those of C. F. Martin and H. A. Lafleur of Montreal. Possibly Osler discussed the subject of the reorganization of the teaching at McGill during the visit of the Montrealers. Osler encouraged Campbell with his hope that "they are beginning to get things settled about the medical school. You keep your mind set on the teaching and the work and do not let practice worry you in the slightest degree. The trouble will be that in a few years you will have more than you can attend to. . . ." In a letter to Marjorie Howard he remarked that everyone believed Campbell would be very successful in Montreal.

In Osler's October 7, 1907, letter to Campbell he mentioned Revere's fishing, swimming and golf lessons during their holiday at Bude in Cornwall, and hoped that Campbell's holiday had also made him "ready for a hard winter's work". He also sent him the initial number of *The Quarterly Journal of Medicine,* of which Archibald Garrod, Humphry Rolleston and Osler were among the editors. However, he commented that the work was being performed by A.G. Gibson, who had just returned from further training by C.G. Schmorl in gross pathology and histology. Thereafter, Gibson took time from his private practice to perform these laboratory duties at the Radcliffe Infirmary.

In Osler's classical description of polycythemia with cyanosis and splenomegaly in 1903, no microscopic studies of the bone marrow were included. He mentioned, however, Vaquez's original 1892 report and hypothesis that the condition might be due to hyperactivity of the hematopoietic organs. Osler's intriguing comment in his January 17, 1908 letter to Campbell, that this disorder "must be a primary bone marrow affair", is a succinct expression of the comments in his lecture of November 28, 1907. He then summarized the findings from six post-mortem examinations: "a plethora vera; intense hyperplasia of the bone marrow, a myelomatosis rubra; and enlargement of the spleen, with histological changes indicative of chronic passive congestion, a uniform hyperplasia of all its elements". Osler discussed haemorrhage and other causes of secondary polycythemia, and continued: "But here is a condition in which, so far as we know, there is an over-supply without any corresponding demand and the same riddle confronts us as in leukaemia and several other diseases of which overproduction of a normal tissue or element is the essence".[68] Researchers today still search for the conclusive answer to this problem.

Osler commissioned Marjorie Howard to purchase a cake for the joint birthday celebrations of Bill Francis and Campbell on April 2, 1908. The Oslers spent October, 1908 through January, 1909 in Paris where Osler studied hard in the libraries and clinics. For his annual Christmas gift to his god-son, he sent pictures of the renowned nineteenth century French physicians, J. N. Corvisart and M.F. X. Bichat. In the accompanying letter, Osler praised the teaching of Joseph Babinski with characteristic comments: "good style precise & accurate. Examines the cases and does not overdo the talking". In his open letters to the *Journal of the American Medical Medical Association* and those to his friends, Osler revealed his admiration of the medical clinics of Professors G. Dieulafoy, F. Raymond, Pierre Marie and Dr. A. Chauffard, his satisfying studies of the works of Michael Servetus and his contemporaries in the 16th century, and the moving experience of his visit to the tomb of his hero, P.C.A. Louis.[69]

In mid-January, the Oslers left Paris to visit the Riviera on the way to Rome where they spent a month. He divided his time between the modern clinics in Rome, Florence, Venice and the other famous centers of North Italy, the historic sights, and the book stalls where he selected many classics for libraries in North America and his own collection. A March postcard to Campbell showed the handsome old lecture room in Bologna. He commented that the clinical work there was excellent and that he reviewed the work in Guido Tizzoni's laboratory on pellagra, a "curious disease". The Italians, of course, had long studied and debated nutritional and environmental factors in this condition. The cause of this disease remained mysterious, however, during Osler's life time and was not known until Joseph Goldberger, Conrad Elvehjem, Tom Spies and their colleagues in America established the nature of the vitamin deficiency. The Oslers left Milan early in April because of important problems concerning new facilities at the Radcliffe Infirmary. Then, after a much anticipated reunion with Revere, and a troublesome confinement with the grippe, Osler sailed with Grace to America on April 21, 1909. Before leaving Montreal on June 18th, he had visited Baltimore, Washington, Philadelphia, New York, Boston, Buffalo, and Toronto, met and inspired many friends and former pupils, advised medical leaders and University Presidents, attended many professional meetings, and given three major addresses.[70]

On May 10, soon after his arrival, he spoke at the Johns Hopkins Historical Club on the life and martyrdom of Michael Servetus, who first described the lesser circulation, and whose four hundredth birth anniversary was being celebrated. Osler had begun the preparation of this manuscript in Paris. He spent many more months to complete it, but it was eventually published.[71]

On May 13, 1909, in the presence of the Governor of Maryland and medical luminaries and representatives of the leading medical libraries, the new building of the Maryland Medical and Chirurgical Faculty was opened with appropriate ceremonies and remarks by prominent people. During the evening meeting to dedicate Osler Hall, he delivered the oration. In this address, "Old and New", he emphasized the importance of all members of the Faculty in devoting themselves, as a united profession, to the public interest.[72] He spent eventful days in several medical centers, including an important gathering with Henry Christian and the medical almuni at Harvard, before visiting his family in Toronto. While in Toronto, he attended the annual meeting of the Ontario Medical Association at which he delivered a notable paper on "The Treatment of Disease". A large crowd of members of the association and visiting physicians, including Campbell Howard, were in attendance. Osler discussed polypharmacy, faith-healing, and other aspects of therapy in words which offered counsel to young practitioners, sympathy and understanding to the older. According to the editor of the *Lancet*, this address earned him "the title of the Nestor of British Medicine".[73]

On the way from the meeting in Toronto, Osler visited his Weston School friend, Ned Milburn in Belleville. He then stayed with the Francis Shepherds and the young Howards in Montreal. After renewing his ties with the McGill College, he sailed for England with Bill Francis and Marjorie Howard.

Marjorie Howard spent the summer months of 1909 with the

Oslers and the Jared Howards in Colonsay. She also became engaged to Osler's former resident and associate, Thomas B. Futcher, whom she had met previously in Baltimore and who came to Oxford for his vacation. According to Osler's well-known advice to young doctors, their attention should be focused on the library and the laboratory before the nursery. Grace and Osler both enjoyed the company of young men and women and encouraged their friendship. There is good evidence to suggest that Osler was not shy about assisting in the matchmaking. Certainly the Oslers brought their nieces and daughters of friends into the company of eligible young men with frequent and happy results. Osler disguised his pleasure by expressing his "desolation" when Amy Gwyn left Oxford to marry his pupil Tom McCrae. He called Marjorie Howard his "Little Missus" in early childhood and a father-daughter relationship between them continued from that time to young adulthood. Both Oslers were delighted when she became engaged to Tom Futcher. Osler's only regret was that the wedding would not take place in Christ Church because they could not be in Montreal on November 24, 1909 to see them walk down the aisle. The newlyweds established their home in Baltimore where T. B. Futcher continued his clinical professorial duties at Johns Hopkins and consultation medical practice.

During the autumn of 1909, Ottilie Wright, a daughter of Osler's friend from McGill student days, began a year at an Oxford school for girls. The Oslers had kept in contact with the Wright family and invited Ottilie frequently to "The Open Arms". She soon joined the family, as if one of Revere's cousins, and helped "Aunt Grace" Osler with the tasks and joys of an assistant hostess for the students and other guests. During the year she acquired a large collection of snapshots of the Osler family and friends at 13 Norham Gardens and the surrounding area. She spent the Christmas Holidays with the Oslers. A feature of the Osler's entertainment for the fourteen year old Revere, the University students and friends, was a large New Year's dance in their house. W. W. Wagstaffe, an undergraduate who later practiced medicine in London and contributed to the Osler Club, and Dinah, a daughter of Osler's niece Isobel Osler Meredith, were among those present. His letter to Marjorie Howard mentioned: "Ottilie is an angel—such a sweet girl and so full of fun—Dinah Meredith is jolly too, when she gets started (Tom kissed them both!) . . ." Osler appears to have enjoyed the party as much as anyone. He was proud of Revere's physical development, but he was anticipating his loneliness after Revere left home for Winchester College on January 19th.[74]

During January, Osler had a recurrence of renal colic, which he had first suffered in 1904. He gave his associate, T. B. Futcher, gravel pebbles in a specimen bottle for diagnostic tests. He apparently mentioned the present attack to ea ʒh of Doctors Thomas, Jacobs, and Futcher. This stone was probably uric acid, but he characteristically jested about his own complaints to Marjorie Futcher on January 25, 1910: "Tell T.B. [Futcher] that the enemy left me yesterday morning (composition C_2H_{10} + $N_{20}S_2$). I had a miserable week but managed to get thro. in fairly good spirits and am thankful it is over. I have had an xray taken to see if this is a quarry, or only diamonds."[75] W. O. was sufficiently recovered within a month to speak at the Samuel Pepys dinner at Cambridge, and prepare his famous Lumelian Lectures on angina pectoris for the Royal College of Physicians during March. Osler had had extensive experience with cardiac disorders as pathologist and physician, and many have considered these lectures among his best clinical descriptions.[76]

Osler regretted that a family illness prevented him from attending the dinner in honor of William Welch in Baltimore. Grace Osler's brother-in-law, Henry Chapin, suddenly became ill with an abdominal sarcoma. She sailed for America on March 20, 1910 and left Osler "in charge of" Ottilie Wright. Even after Grace returned on April 19, Ottilie stayed to help their niece, Nona Gwyn, entertain the frequent visitors to "The Open Arms". In Osler's letter to Marjorie at this time he told of Revere's happiness at Winchester and fishing for trout during the holidays in Wales.[77] He also mentioned that sweet Ottilie would make "a good wife for old Campbell", and quickly consoled the pregnant Marjorie: "But how I wish you could be here! No one can take your place & we miss you horribly."

CHAPTER IV

Changes of Medicine at Iowa and The Hopkins

DURING THE YEARS since Campbell Howard had returned to Montreal, Osler kept up with the local situation and encouraged him with approval of his activities. He cited reports of Campbell's fine clinics at the Montreal General Hospital, and assured him that the young faculty doctors and students supported him. In his letter of April 25, 1910, he mentioned that he was sending reprints of his Lumelian Lectures on angina, and recent books by Ludwig Aschoff on pathological anatomy and by Franz Hamburger on tuberculosis in children. He also remarked: "You certainly seem to have your hands full with teaching. We all hear your work is telling and you are getting a splendid grip on the students, and evidently there is no one in medicine in the running, either in Montreal or in the country, and I am sure you are close to the reward of all of your hard work. I suppose you are certain of the wards at the next vacancy at the [Montreal] General." Campbell's current clinical duties were confined to the "out-door" department rather than the wards, but senior physicians, such as F. G. Finley, often provided their in-patients for his studies. Osler did not mention in his letter a possible offer to Campbell from the University of Iowa, but he may have heard of it through his contacts with Abraham Flexner or William Welch. Welch had long been an advisor to the Rockefeller Institute and Foundation, and was the recognized leader of medical science and education. He was elected president of the American Medical Association in 1909, and stressed in his

Presidential address in April, 1910 the progress towards higher standards of medical education. After their first professional contacts, he and Abraham Flexner respected each other and the younger man modeled many of his recommendations on the ideas of Welch and the success of the Johns Hopkins development.[78]

In the latter decades of the 19th century, efforts to reform medical education were started by the American Medical Association, together with the Association of American Medical Colleges and various state licensing boards. These efforts made little headway until the 1902 reorganization of the AMA. Then the successful recruitment of members in affiliated local societies across the nation greatly increased its strength in representing the medical profession. Its Council on Medical Education, under Chairman Arthur D. Bevan, began to function in 1904, and Dr. N. P. Colwell became the first secretary. Standards were set to classify more than 160 American medical colleges, and during 1906–07 a representative visited and inspected each school. After receiving their evaluations some agreed to improve their curricula and others planned to consolidate or disband, but some medical and political groups protested that the AMA was motivated by self-interest.

The Carnegie Foundation for the Advancement of Teaching had earned the public trust for its handling of endowments for teachers in North American colleges. Its officers recognized the great variability of the standards and organization of the colleges, universities and associated professional schools. Often schools of law or medicine were not adequately supported or controlled. The objectives of institutions in the fields of education and medicine coincided and talented men were available. In December, 1908, President Henry S. Pritchett and Mr. Abraham Flexner represented the Carnegie Foundation in deliberations with medical leaders and their study was begun. The Carnegie Foundation officers acknowledged the cooperation of the Council on Education of the American Medical Association, the secretary of the Association of American Colleges, William H. Welch of Johns Hopkins University, and Simon Flexner of the Rockefeller Institute. Simon was Abraham Flexner's brother, and both he and Welch knew the established teachers and their promising pupils in the leading medical institutions. By February, 1910, Abraham Flexner, often accompanied by a medical colleague, had visited every teaching institution. He had completed his detailed report for publication by April, 1910.[79]

Abraham Flexner visited the McGill College of Medicine in March, before two trips to Iowa during 1909. The original draft of his opinion distressed many of the medical faculty and members of the Iowa State Board of Education. Accordingly, W. R. Boyd, Chairman of the Board's Finance Committee, arranged with President Pritchett of the Carnegie Foundation to have Mr. Flexner return to Iowa City. He arrived in November, 1909, in the company of R. H. Whitehead, M.D., Dean of Medicine, University of Virginia. The original report was confirmed and presented to the Iowa State Board of Education on December 10, 1909. The report was mentioned, but not filed with the minutes of the Board. Recently, however, an undated typescript was located among President G. E. MacLean's correspondence in an appropriate file for the medical college. The signature was typed and several spelling errors remained uncorrected. The following text is more detailed than the published version.

STATE UNIVERSITY OF IOWA. MEDICAL DEPARTMENT. [COLLEGE]

The medical department of the State University of Iowa must be considered in two sections. The equipment and instruction in the scientific branches occupying the first two years are generally good and in some points excellent. The work in anatomy is admirable. A better equipped department, more enthusiastically conducted, is hardly to be found anywhere in the country. There is unmistakable evidence of excellent teaching and intelligent scientific activity. To some extent, the same may be said of physiology, pathology, bacteriology, and other fundamental branches, though these departments have been less generously treated in the way of skilled assistants. The men in charge of them are, however, zealous and energetic; their ideals high, and the equipment in the shape of apparatus and books, modern and sufficient.

The clinical situation is of a different order altogether. In the first place, it lacks the close correlation which the scientific departments have achieved. The executive officer [Guthrie] of the department lives at Dubuque and comes to Iowa City two days weekly. The professor of surgery [Jepson] resides at Sioux City. It is clear that under these conditions the clinical side cannot develop as a unit, nor can there grow up between the scientific men and the partly non-resident clinicians the close interrelation char-

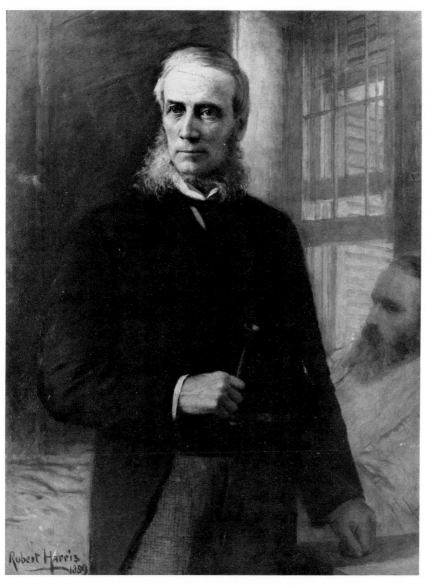

1.   Robert Palmer Howard, M.D.

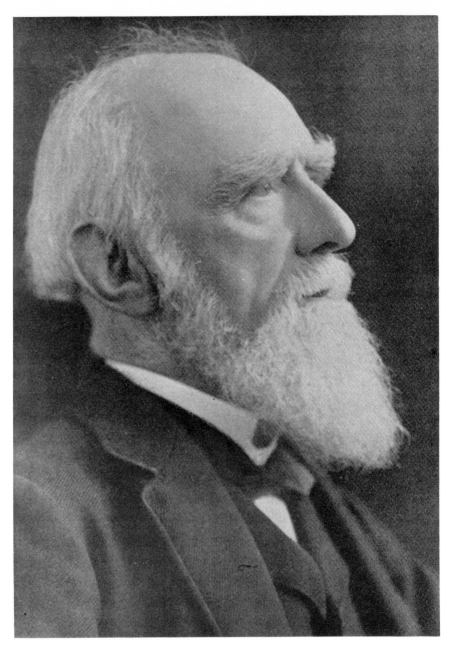

2.   Lord Strathcona

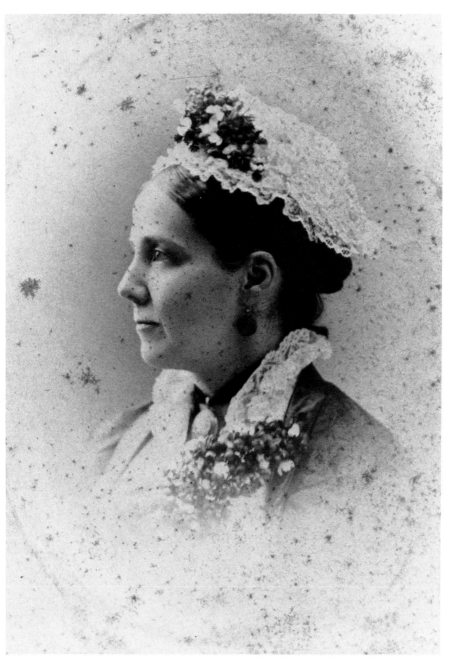

3.   Emily Severs Howard

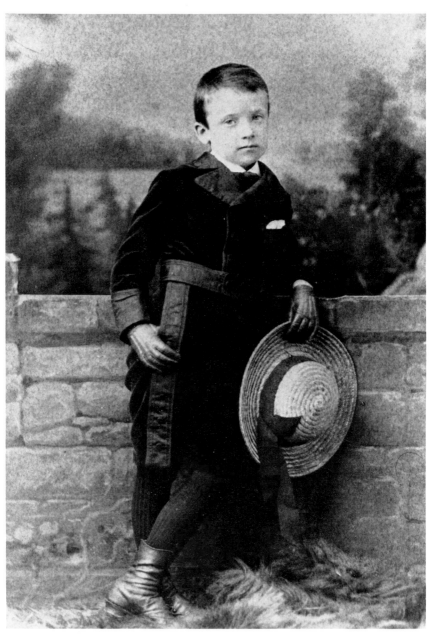

4.   Campbell P. Howard, age 6, 1883

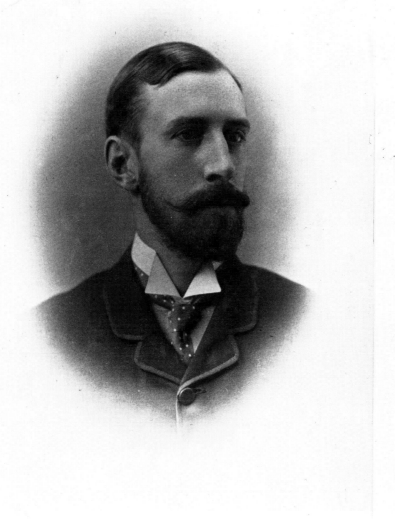

5.   Robert Jared Bliss Howard, M.D.

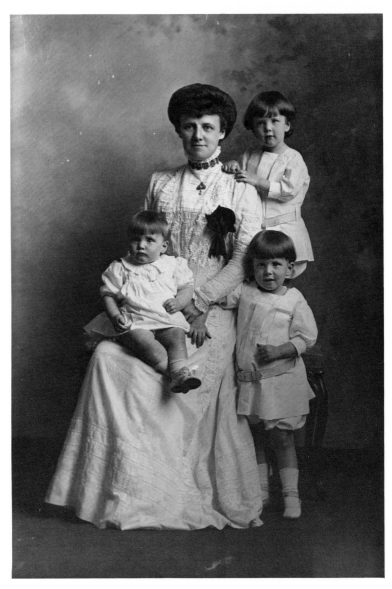

6.   Muriel Howard Eberts, with Edmond (behind),
      Beatrice (on her lap, and Hermann, July 7, 1909

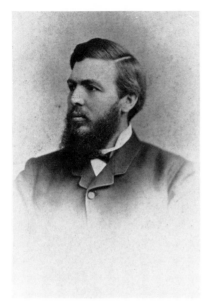

7. Henry P. Wright, M.D.

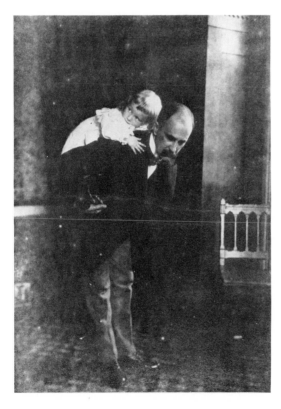

8. Osler and Revere, age 2

Campbell Howard
with the author's
love
aug. 2 6th
1898.

THE PRINCIPLES AND
PRACTICE OF MEDICINE

DESIGNED FOR THE USE OF PRACTITIONERS
AND STUDENTS OF MEDICINE

BY

WILLIAM OSLER, M. D.

Fellow of the Royal Society ; Fellow of the Royal College of Physicians,
London ; Professor of Medicine in the Johns Hopkins University and
Physician-in-chief to the Johns Hopkins Hospital, Baltimore ;
formerly Professor of the Institutes of Medicine, McGill
University, Montreal ; and Professor of Clinical Medicine
in the University of Pennsylvania, Philadelphia

THIRD EDITION

NEW YORK
D. APPLETON AND COMPANY
1898

9.   Title page inscribed to Campbell Howard

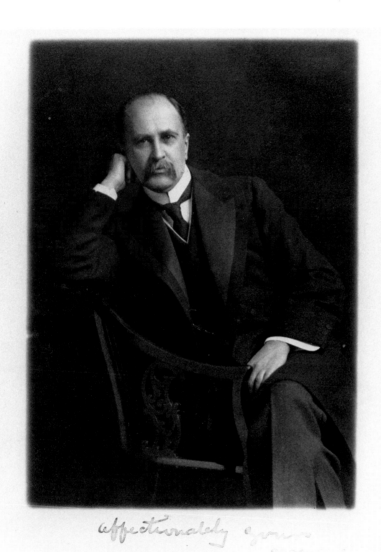

10. *Affectionately yours Wm. Osler,* c. 1902

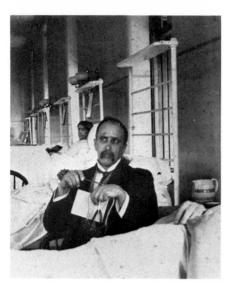

11.   *Dr. Osler*

12.   *Dr. Osler's Ward Rounds*

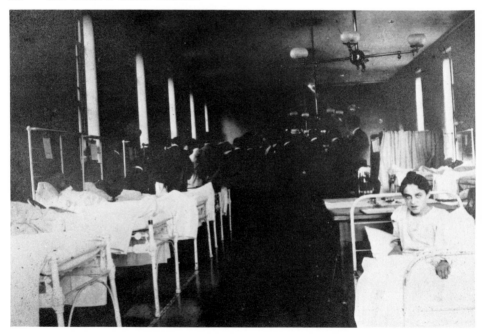

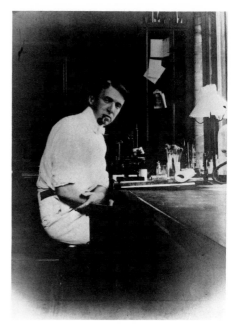

13.   Campbell P. Howard, 1903

14.   Staff, Dept. of Medicine, Johns Hopkins Hospital, 1903–04

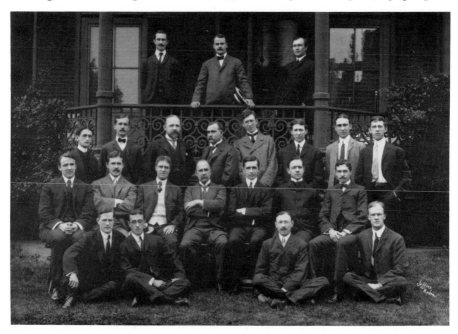

THE PRINCIPLES AND PRACTICE OF MEDICINE

*DESIGNED FOR THE USE OF PRACTITIONERS
AND STUDENTS OF MEDICINE*

BY

WILLIAM OSLER, M. D.

FELLOW OF THE ROYAL SOCIETY; FELLOW OF THE ROYAL COLLEGE OF PHYSICIANS,
LONDON; REGIUS PROFESSOR OF MEDICINE, OXFORD UNIVERSITY; HONORARY PRO-
FESSOR OF MEDICINE, JOHNS HOPKINS UNIVERSITY, BALTIMORE; FORMERLY
PROFESSOR OF THE INSTITUTES OF MEDICINE, McGILL UNIVERSITY,
MONTREAL; AND PROFESSOR OF CLINICAL MEDICINE IN THE
UNIVERSITY OF PENNSYLVANIA, PHILADELPHIA

*SIXTH EDITION, THOROUGHLY REVISED
FROM NEW PLATES*

NEW YORK AND LONDON
D. APPLETON AND COMPANY
1905

15.–16. Presentation copy of Sixth Edition, inscribed *Dr. Campbell Howard from Wm. Osler*

PRESENTATION COPY

This is Number __ *19*

of the first 105,000 copies printed

Dr Campbell Howard

from

Wm Osler

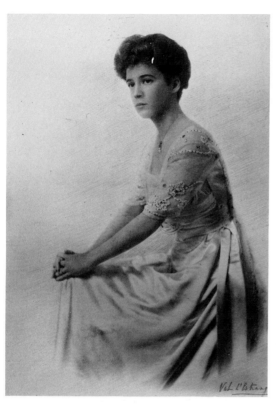

17.   Marjorie Howard, c. 1905

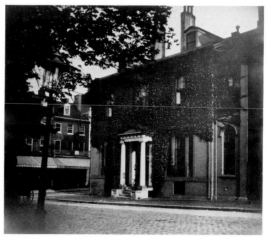

18.   Number 1 West Franklin Street

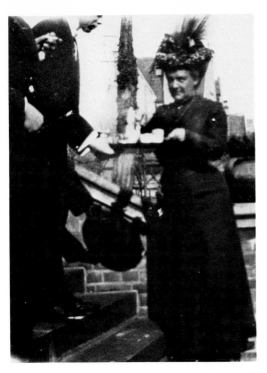

19.   Grace Osler as the
hostess of *The Open
Arms,* c. 1910
20.   Three Oslers, Oxford,
June 1905

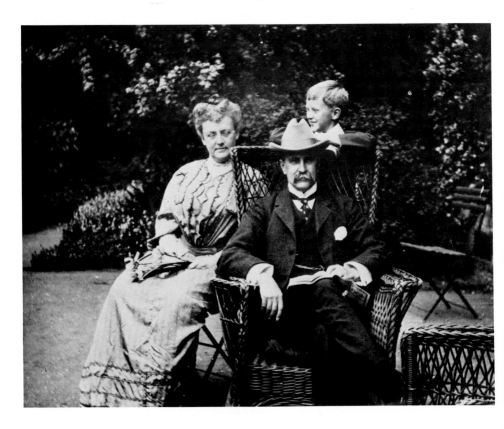

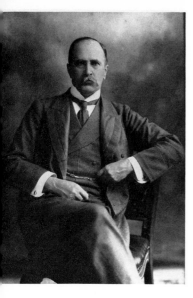

21.   William Osler, c. 1907

22.   Osler, 13 Norham Gardens, c. 1910

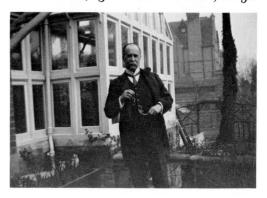

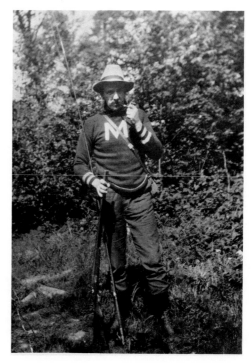

23.   C.P. Howard at a camp in the
Province of Quebec, c.1910

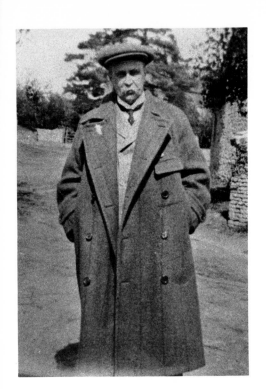
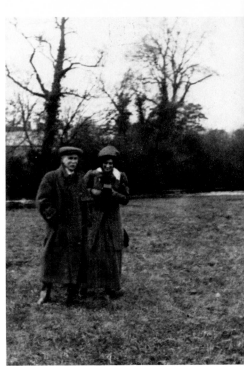

24–26. An Easter outing on the Coln, Fairford, Gloucester, April 17, 1910; Osler, Osler and Ottilie Wright, Revere and Dr. W.J. Turrell

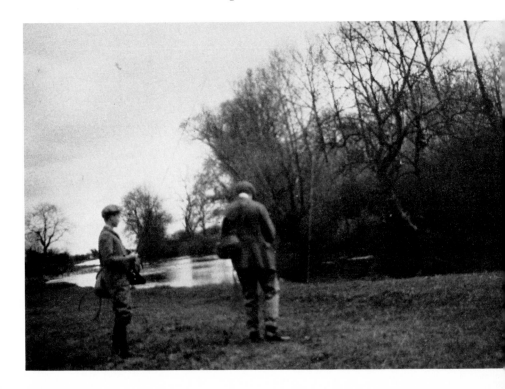

acteristic of a medical department that functions as a whole.

Facts confirm this criticism. The clinical instruction is given in the University Hospital, in which less than 90 beds are available for teaching purposes. With the question as to how far the actual needs of clinical teaching can be met by this number of beds, I shall deal later. The point now is that the conduct of the hospital, as a teaching adjunct, reflects just the disorganization above hinted at. The hospital is, in its teaching aspects, headless. President MacLean witnessed my unavailing efforts to find anyone— nurse or physician—who could describe the system on which the bedside teaching was conducted. There are, for example, no hospital records worthy the name. No hospital report has been compiled. It is impossible to say what ground the clinical teaching has actually covered, just as it is impossible succinctly to describe what takes place in the way of clinical discipline. Now, as the technique of clinical teaching is in these days quite definite, the conclusion is irresistible that vagueness indicates unorganized and more or less antiquated methods of teaching. One of the clnical men admitted frankly "boys don't follow medical cases as closely as they might."

The inference fairly to be made from the preceding facts is sustained by the dispensary. The only records are notes in a book. I was told that at the close of the year a card index would be compiled; but just where complete data for this index were to come from or why it should be made at the close of the year or what its character or use was to be, I could not learn. The eye and ear clinic is large; the medical clinic is small. There are no clinics in surgery, gynecology, or G-U.

Now there are two points of view from which to survey the preceding situation:

1. Taking the clinical opportunities as they stand, they are not used for all they are worth; nor can they be so used, until a resident dean, a resident clinical faculty, and a hospital superintendent familiar with the technique of modern medical teaching are secured. It is necessary at once to adopt a more adequate form of taking case histories and keeping case records; the students must be trained to be parts of the hospital in its primary function of curing diseases, and the records of every case should at every stage indicate what the student has seen and done and how it has been checked up or controlled by interne, staff officer and professor, so that the complete record may regularly form the basis of conference and discussion. It is obvious that this involves increasing

expense at the start, though the point I have thus far emphasized is more *organization* of what already exists.

2. It is doubtful, however, whether, even if the foregoing policy is pursued, the school will become clinically adequate. There are 100 students in the third and fourth years. They have access to less than 90 beds. This is much too little for general medicine and surgery, and yet it includes everything that the clinical teachers of all departments can use. Some branches, e. g., infectious diseases are altogether omitted. Post-mortem work is far too limited. In obstetrics there were last year 45 cases available; this year "not so many." Yet a senior class of 50 students—the present enrollment—ought to have at least 250 obstetric cases. It is thus absolutely indisputable that more clinical material and of greater variety must be obtained.

To this increase, the local condition is not readily favorable. On the other hand, it may be at once conceded that indefinite increase of clinical material is not essential, and may prove embarassing. Granted a barely adequate supply, the thoroughness with which it is used to train a small body of students in painstaking methods of studying and handling their cases may more than outweigh a few deficiencies.

To sum up:

Iowa fails to provide clinical training of high technical quality; it fails to supply an adequate supply of material. These defects can perhaps both be remedied by the formation of a really eminent faculty which, reinforced by liberal state support, will probably draw to Iowa City all the clinical material that is needed; and by the same token, such a faculty would promptly reconstruct the clinical teaching. There is thus presented a fairly sharp alternative; the clinical teaching can be improved without any greater expenditure than is involved in securing a permanent resident surgeon, and a hospital head. But these steps will not of themselves cure the fundamental difficulty. That calls for an enlarged hospital, an increased and expensive faculty. Is it worthwhile to take the first step unless in the near future Iowa will be ready to take the second? And considering its present opportunities for expansion in other directions, on which no natural handicap is imposed, is it wise educational statesmanship to endeavor, against the grave obstacles inherent in the situation, to develop a department which will in every stage consume an ever increasing proportion of the resources of the University? A proper provision for medical education in centers of population like Chicago and Minneapolis is proving a heavy load to carry. Far heavier, of course, will be a satisfactory provision in a small inland residential community; and in view of the fact that a decided reduction in the number of medical schools is called for, it is worth considering whether the general interest, educational and social, will not best be served by a differentiation which in the future will limit medical training to institutions in large centers plus perhaps one or two like Ann Arbor, already so highly developed that just now it costs less to go on than to stop. These considerations ought to be carefully weighted by institutions that, now comparatively undeveloped on the clinical side, must contemplate in the near future a large expenditure on that score, if they persist.

Three institutions whose experience is of suggestive value to Iowa at this crisis may be cited;

Ann Arbor, already alluded to, where a really admirable department has been developed at great expense, and during a time when the general level of clinical instruction was low. Now, however, that this level has risen, Ann Arbor feels keenly the competition of institutions more favorably located, so that, despite its great start, the question of the future of its clinical department gives rise to serious concern. There is little doubt that if the clinical department were at this moment relatively undeveloped, the institution would hesitate to embark on its development now.

Madison, where, despite local opportunities greatly superior to Iowa City, the University has contentedly limited itself to two years' work.

Missouri, where, in a situation analogous to Iowa City, the regents confronted with a choice between greatly augmented expenditure on clinical medicine or abandoning it altogether, have just chosen the latter alternative and have chosen to discontinue the clinical department.

In deciding a similar question, Iowa must, in addition to considerations already started, reflect that its present clinical department—100 strong—is on a high school basis and has grown up in competition with the hitherto weak clinical schools of the west. A year or more hence two years of college work are to be required for entrance in the college of medicine. This change will greatly reduce numbers. Simultaneously a much more critical attitude with reference to clinical opportunities is growing, and students better trained in fundamental branches will be in a position to distinguish between real and half-way clinical opportunities. So far there has been perhaps little to choose between. But in the near future certainly Minneapolis and probably Chicago will furnish clinical instruction that will crowd schools of inadequate clinical resources very hard. It would seem inevitable that to hold its own in such a competition will prove an increasingly disproportionate burden on the income of any institution laboring, on account of location, under grave disadvantages.

Abraham Flexner.[80]

Flexner's report was referred to the Faculty Committee of the Board of Education and the Dean of Medicine for action. Walter L. Bierring resigned the Chair of Medicine at Iowa University to be Professor of Medicine at Drake University College of Medicine and practice in Des Moines.[81] At the meetings of May 25–26, 1910, the Board approved the plan to reorganize the Medical College, and enlarge the hospital to include more clinical and private beds and additional laboratories. The Board then invited Abraham Flexner to return to Iowa City to give further detailed suggestions regarding the building and the selection of personnel. He recommended the establishment of a clinical research laboratory, and the appointment of a clinician with modern training to head the department of theory and practice of medicine. He suggested several, including Campbell P. Howard, for consideration.[82]

Campbell Howard visited the University of Iowa during the summer of 1910 regarding the vacancy as Head of the Department. He appreciated the ability of several faculty members including Assistant Professor Clarence Van Epps. However, he considered that it would be difficult to develop a department which provided good clinical instruction, and also undertook new studies in clinical research. The May, 1910, budget included $4,000 per year for the professor of medicine and $1,500 for one assistant professor, but it was inadequate for laboratory apparatus and salary for a research assistant. Negotiations were continued through a second visit to Iowa City. Late in July, the Medical Faculty selected Campbell Howard. The Finance Committee of the Board was authorized to complete financial arrangements with him so that he would start in September, 1910. Campbell Howard and W. R. Boyd, who played the key administrative role in the budgetary discussions, soon formed a mutual respect and trust. This was important for the successful establishment of the medical department and the further development of the College of Medicine. In his July 29 letter to Howard, President MacLean included the privilege to nominate a second assistant at a salary of $1,500 for the first year, and a fund of $750 for equipment. Howard's reply on August 3 raised questions about the details of the budget for the running expenses and equipment of the clinical research laboratory. A notation was made that Boyd answered the questions. Campbell Howard continued on August 3: "I leave tomorrow for Quebec to have a chat with Dr. Osler, who arrives from England. After my chat with him I will forward you my official acceptance. If he approves of my going to Iowa City, as I feel certain he will, I will write you my official letter. I plan to arrive in Iowa City about two weeks before the opening of the session—in time to get things in running order. Please accept my thanks for your courtesy and kindness to me in these negotiations. I trust that I will be able to fulfill the expectations you and Dean [J. R.] Guthrie entertain for me. Also that you will always be interested in the Medical School and will continue to aid us all in placing the department at the head of the Medical Schools of the Middle West. . . ."[83]

How frequently Campbell had consulted W. Osler during these negotiations is not known, but a cable late in July prompted W. O. to write Principal Peterson of McGill on July 28:

"I had a cable from Campbell Howard last night saying that he had practically accepted the Professorship of medicine at the University of Ohio [Iowa]. This is one of the many outcomes of the Carnegie report; they have reorganized the medical department of the University. While I am very sorry that he is leaving Montreal, in many ways it will be a good thing for him to have an independent position, and it is sure to be a stepping-stone to a chair in one of the big universities. Campbell has a great grip on the men of his own standing, and the students are always devoted to him. I never had a more satisfactory assistant, and he has splendid ideals. It has been uphill work for him in Montreal, though I have always been confident that he would do well; he is a great loss to the school and country".

Principal Peterson replied to Osler on September 24, 1910,:

". . . I ought also to refer to your letter of 28th July about Campbell Howard. I wrote to him at once and had a very pleasant letter from him in reply. His departure is probably inevitable, but you may rely upon us to keep our eye on him and to get him back if we can. Will you write to me if there is anything that I can do or if you have any advice to offer? . . ."[84]

Grace, Revere and Osler left England on July 29 on the *Empress of Ireland* with Ottilie Wright and Nona Gwyn, and they reached Quebec on Thursday, August 4, 1910. Before docking,

Osler included in his letter to Marjorie Futcher: "I am greatly excited about Campbell's offer & he has cabled that he thinks of accepting. It will be a great temptation to get his own clinique and it will only be a stepping stone to something better. I hope he may be at Quebec tomorrow, but these trips may have taken so much time that he cannot get away." Campbell met the boat and discussed the Iowa situation with his mentor before he telegraphed his final acceptance to President MacLean.

Grace and W. Osler relaxed for nearly two weeks at Murray Bay. Campbell had often gone fishing during the summer with Frank Ross of Quebec. Revere spent the first week trout-fishing with the two men at Ross' camp, "Tantari", which was about 40 miles north of Quebec. Osler's satisfaction with Campbell's new appointment is shown in his letter to H. B. Jacobs, as well as the following on August 8, 1910 to Campbell:

"The more I think of it the better I am pleased with the Iowa prospect. There will be many small worries & difficulties, but you can do a good bit of work & stir up matters medical in that region. I leave here next Sunday eve & will bring my things to your house. If [F.J.] Shepherd is at Como I shall spend the night there. I go on to Toronto next Tuesday eve [August 16]. We can have time for a good talk. There are a number of things to go over. I hope you & Ike have had a good time. It is most kind of you to have given him this great pleasure."[85]

While Campbell prepared to move to his new post, the Oslers visited many relatives and friends in Canada and in Northeastern American cities and summer resorts. Osler was about to sail from New York on September 6, when he sent Campbell a note with expressions of cheer, encouragement and help:

"Welcome to the west—to your new home & duties. There will be many worries & things will not turn out as you wish always but a quiet tongue & a smile will help. As Harvey C. said this position puts you & the man [A.W. Hewlett] at Ann Arbor in the running for the next good berth. I will get the slides ready for you—useful for p.g. [postgraduate] lectures or outside semi-popular ones. Tommy and A.G. [Grace] send love. Write soon. I had a nice letter from [President] MacLean."

While Campbell was settling in to his new responsibility in Iowa, Marjorie and T. B. Futcher's first child was born on September 13, 1910. The child was named after his grandfather, Palmer Howard, but not Thomas as Osler had suggested. Osler was pleased to be a god father. In his September 17 letter to Campbell, he also noted that he had written leading doctors in Chicago, and that Grace Osler had written a cousin in Iowa about Campbell's arrival. He urged Campbell to continue his public education efforts against tuberculosis as he had in Montreal as the director of the St. George's Tuberculosis Class:

"We got back safely after a very good trip. We had a cable the day before yesterday about Palmer Howard Futcher, which was very good news. You will have a hard time I know to get settled. I have written today to [Frank] Billings, [James B.] Herrick, [Arthur R.] Edwards, [Henry B.] Favill, and [Ludvig] Hektoen of Chicago, so that you can write or call upon any one of them, they will know about you. Grace has written to the Perkins of Burlington who are delightful people. Your experience with the tuberculosis work in Montreal will be most helpful, you could spend a little time stumping the country in the cause. I will have the lantern slides copied and will send the books. They will have to go by freight; I am afraid the parcel will be too big for the Smithsonian."

The reference to the large books was to the *Revue de Médecine*. Campbell eventually obtained this set, presumably from the "Chief", along with many reprints. His collection of unbound articles by Osler eventually numbered over 400 items, and was particularly strong in the clinical medicine and literary publications from the Baltimore and Oxford periods.

In an October, 1910, letter to Marjorie he mentioned their happiness about her son and other family news, and included a generous comparison with his own teacher: "Campbell writes most enthusiastically—he will own the State within a year. He can teach like your father & he has his capacity for hard work." This preceded Osler's October 20 letter to Campbell:

"It was very nice to have your letter and to hear such good accounts of the work. I knew you would be busy as a bee from the start; you will have difficulty in finding time for your work. I am getting the slides ready; they will go next week by the American express. Some of them I am afraid have faded a bit. The set showing the rashes in infectious diseases will be most useful; I have forgotten who sent them from Cleveland to me, but they make a stunning set for demonstration of the rashes. The abdominal tumours will do for outside lectures . . ."

Osler's letters for the next three months concerned sending materials for Campbell's teaching. He acknowledged the receipt of several long letters about Campbell's experiences at Iowa, but copies unfortunately are not available. Osler also mentioned Revere going to dances and accompanying his parents to the theater in London. In a letter to Marjorie Futcher he remarked: "We are saving to buy a farm for Isaac [Revere]. He will never do anything at books. He has grown so much & is very happy, but I doubt if Winchester is the place for him as there is nothing but classics." The farm was never purchased, but the father repeatedly expressed his concern about Revere's difficulties with the Latin and Greek languages.

Early in January, 1911, the Oslers were grieved by a cable from Bill Francis's sister, Marian Osborne, that he had tuberculosis, which was later described as a small spot at the apex of one lung. He was treated by J. Roddick Byers at the sanatorium at Ste. Agathe in the Laurentian Mountains until August, 1912. Though his health recovered, he did not return to medical practice, but took the position of general secretary of the Canadian Medical Association and assistant editor of its *Journal*. At that time Osler remarked in a letter to Marjorie Futcher that this work "would give him a small salary and literary duties which he likes. I fear he is not cut out for the rough and tumble of practice." Osler, of course, would not be alive to share in the praise of his kinsman's success as editor of the *Bibliotheca Osleriana*, and curator of the Osler Library at McGill.

Osler's match-making propensities are amusingly illustrated in the letter to Marjorie January 15, 1911, shortly after Campbell had visited the Futchers: "I wish he would marry that Perkins girl. G. [Grace] says she is a peach. Revere says Nona [Gwyn] would not do as she could not go fishing with him. That gem Ottilie is too young, tho. she is a treasure and we are devoted to her." A few months later the match would be made. In the meantime Campbell worked hard at Iowa City and, while Grace Osler in Oxford kept a maternal eye on Revere at Winchester, Osler left Oxford on February 4 to join his brother Edmund Osler's party in Egypt.

Campbell Howard received cards with scenes of Cairo, an obelisk at Luxor and the ruins of the great hall at Karnak. On February 20, 1911, in a letter to Marjorie Futcher, Osler gave many details of the journey up the Nile in the chartered launch, *Seti:*

"Here I am on a great spree—only I wish you & the baby were here in this glorious sunshine. This is a beauty—boat holds six or eight—everything furnished & found by T.C. [Thomas Cook] & son. A big burly dragoman is in charge and there is a crew of 30 all told—two cooks, a laundry man, three waiters & every luxury. E.B.O. [Sir Edmund Boyd Osler], Mrs. Wilmot Matthews (Amo), her husband, Elsie Bethune & Ernest Cattanach form the party

(Fig. 28). We shall go as far as Assouan, 580 miles & then come back slowly seeing the sights on the way. It takes a month. It is too bad that G. [Grace] could not come, but she would not have felt happy both so far away from Ike. We are four or five days without stopping at any post-office. We tie up at night to a bank, anywhere. Yesterday we had our first excursion to the rock tombs of Beni-Hasan—only 800 of them some as big as a church & all dug out of the solid rock. Walls covered with colored sketches & hieroglyphics. I wish you could have seen us start out on donkeys surrounded by an admiring crowd of Egyptians. Cairo was fascinating—full of old friends. There were twenty Canadians whom we knew at Shepheards [Hotel]. It is a new sensation to be travelling *au prince* [in royal style], and no bills to pay. . . . Our Capt. is a direct descendant of Ramses II, same face, identical profile. There is an extraordinary persistence of this Egyptian type. The dragoman is an Arab, but looks more like a fat Turk. Fortunately he talks English well and knows the river thoroughly. It has been very cold. Yesterday I wore my fur coat. I never remember sitting a whole day in it before. Today is gorgeous 68 & no wind. We stick in a mud bank every few hours & have to be poled off. Yesterday we tried to help an express steamer which had been aground 24 hrs but we broke our steering gear in the attempt & were delayed 6 hours. The crops are just coming up & we pass long stretches of the most brilliant green—wheat, onions [and] beans seem the chief crop, but they grow much cotton & sugar cane. The factory chimneys show the prosperity of the country—rarely out of sight. English everywhere. How mad the French must be to be supplanted in this way, but it was their own fault."

Beginning in the 29th century B.C., the Tombs of Beni-Hasan were made for feudal nobles of the 4th and 5th dynasties. Priests were in charge of preserving these tombs. They were restored and modified during the time of Queen Hatshepsut in the 15th century B.C. Ramses II was a powerful pharoah whose handsome appearance is preserved in a black granite statue.[86]

On March 18, the launch returned to Cairo where Osler spent a few more days. His Egyptian experiences led to revisions of the descriptions of several tropical diseases in the 8th edition of the textbook. He also mentioned the prevalence of typhoid fever, tuberculosis, bilharziasis and anklyostomiasis in the Nile Valley in several letters.[87]

At the end of March, Osler visited Italy, spending several days in Pompeii, Sorrento and other places near Naples. Campbell had apparently reported his concerns about sectarians and poor standards of practice. At that time, the homeopathic practitioners were vociferously campaigning to gain public support against plans to consolidate with the Medical College, and eventually eliminate the University of Iowa College of Homeopathic Medicine. The Still College of Osteopathy at Des Moines, though condemned by Flexner, continued in operation. Osler referred to articles in the lay press, which exposed abuses in all the health professions, and concluded that the past performance of the regular physicians was partly responsible for the present situation. Osler also mentioned activities which would take place in June in his letter from Naples on March 28, 1911:

"One of your letters must have gone astray—not unlikely as I have been wandering very far afield. Bill [Francis] seems doing well. . . . I have just had yours of Feb. 27th. sent on from Assouan! We missed several batches of letters on the Nile. The trip has been a wonderful one—so many new impressions. Cairo is a fascinating city. I saw good deal of [Llewellyn] Phillips & of the work at the [Kasr-el-Ainy] Hospital. But they need reorganization—complete & through. If Germany had the country for about 2 years, it would do the Egyptians good & their drastic measures would put the educational system in order. The Ross' asked after you. James R. has been very ill—pressure symptoms increasing upon his windpipe & rt. bronchus—very remarkable case. I saw him 7 years ago with Arthur Browne when he had a simple aortic insuff. Now there must be dil. [dilatation] of the arch. No physical signs of aneurism. I know how galling the conditions must be but great heavens they are mending. A section of the public at any rate is awake. Such crusades as have been carried on by the Ladies Home Journal and by the Colliers Weekly must do good. We are ourselves suffering for the sins of the fathers. No standard was set for generations and there was no difference between the training of a regular physician and the others. It is often discouraging, but I am sure the outlook is improving. When are you coming over? I should like to meet you somewhere in the continent, tho. after this long holiday I must stay at home & mind the shop. I will arrange for the Journal [Quarterly J. of Medicine] nos. to be sent. I have them. Fortunately we are doing well with it—far better than we had expected. . . . Nona [Gwyn] & Ottilie will come over again & the Coronation will bring many friends. I hear that Dr. [H.M.] Hurd has resigned. 'Twas time. He has had a good long spell & the work is now too heavy. I wish I could get out to the McGill opening [of the new medical building] but it is impossible. June is my very busy month —exams &c. I enclose two photos of the Nile trip."[(88)]

The next letters mentioned that Maude Abbott was in bed at "The Open Arms," recovering from a sore leg, and that Revere now was taller than his Father, and had had little success while deep-sea fishing because of rough weather at Tenby, Wales. Osler also asked for notes and corrections from Campbell for the next edition of his textbook.

During May, 1911, discussions about the changes proposed in the clinical departments at Baltimore worried Osler. The General Education Board of the Rockefeller philanthropies, under the influence of Dr. William H. Welch and Abraham Flexner, was considering awarding funds to Johns Hopkins University to establish whole-time professors for several clinical departments. Osler's concerns about the wisdom of this plan were expressed in his letters to his former Baltimore colleagues, Professor W. S. Thayer on June 22, and H. A. Kelly on August 25, 1911. His more detailed letter to President I.D. Remsen, intended for the consideration of the Johns Hopkins faculty, was sent early in September, 1911.[89]

After the General Education Board's announcement in 1913 that it had given $1,500,000 to fund the new plan at Johns Hopkins Medical School, Osler accepted the development with mixed feelings. In a published comment, Osler expressed gratification that the name of his friend, William H. Welch, was associated with the endowment. Osler informed Welch about this note in advance so that his response could be published in the next issue.[90]

He referred to the Hopkins situation, as well as an unfulfilled plan to join Campbell in Berlin, as he emphasized by asterisks in the letter of May 23, 1911: "It will be splendid to see you the end of July. Come directly here from Plymouth.* You must have had a strenuous winter, but it has been a novel and interesting experience. That is a good letter-paper-heading. What a busy time they are having in Baltimore trying to settle the question of whole-time Professors. There is much to be said on both sides. I have not had any details, but the figures mentioned by [H.A.] Kelly, 7500 dollars, would of course be absurd: but $15–20,000 would do. A. G. [Grace] tells me that you are going to Germany first.* Let me know when you are to be in Berlin, I should like so much to get a chance to have a few days there with you. I hope your boys will do well in the examination."

Many ceremonies were held in connection with the Coronation of King George V and Queen Mary in London. Grace, soon to be Lady Osler, was accompanied by the youthful Nona Gwyn and Ottilie Wright at their presentation to the Court, all of them dressed in suitably fashionable attire. Photographs showed that the elder woman's handsome appearance was scarcely excelled by the flush of youthful beauty (Figs. 29 and 32). Osler's preoccupations caused him to avoid most of the celebrations, but on June 20, 1911, *The Times* (London) included his name on the list of those to receive a Baronetcy. The following day he wrote Marjorie Futcher:

"What do you think of Sir Billy? How I wish you were here— to squeeze & Palmer. Such times! We knew ten days ago. Asquith [Prime Minister] wrote that the King intended to confer a Baronetcy of the United Kingdom upon me. We could of course say nothing. Yesterday the lists were out, & the telegrams have been raining in fast ever since—nearly fifty cables from the other side. Of course we are pleased. Living here these things mean a great deal, but nothing could add to our happiness. Personally I have had more than my share of these honours. How I wish your father was alive! Campbell cabled. We shall hope to see him before long. We have been over heads & ears in all sorts of engagements— chiefly floaters who come in. I have been a great deal in town [London] & Grace & the girls have done so much. You will be enchanted with her presentation picture—splendid! Could not be better. Ike is a bit overwhelmed as the boys immediately began to call him Sir Revere. You would not know him—1/2 an inch taller than his dad. He is really a dear boy, but Latin- & Greek-less. Still, no matter, he has a good heart."[91]

Osler continued to be busy with his writing and other professional duties. Campbell agreed to join him at the British Medical Association meeting in Birmingham which began on July 25, 1911. Osler discussed W. Hale White's paper at the Section of Medicine on "The Diagnosis of Fever Without Physical Signs", and T. C. Fox's paper at the Dermatology Section on "The Vascular Disorders of the Skin and Their Relation to Other Morbid States". Osler was one of the speakers at "The Discussion of Administrative Control of Tuberculosis". There he supported the development of tuberculosis dispensaries in association with general hospitals and county infirmaries. He and Campbell met "many nice fellows".[92]

Campbell Howard and Osler arrived at the front steps of "The Open Arms" on July 27 or 28 where Grace, Nona Gwyn and Ottilie Wright were awaiting them. The thirty-three year-old professor fell in love with the eighteen year-old Ottilie at first sight. Lady Osler had already planned to go in advance of Osler and Revere to a summer resort at Llanddulas in North Wales. Campbell chose to accompany the three ladies. He became engaged on August 9 to "a maid that paragons perfection", to cite Osler's quotation from Shakespeare.[93] Marjorie Futcher was with her sister, Muriel, at a Canadian seaside village when Osler wrote her on August 10, the day he reached Llanddulas. "Such excitement in the household! I am perfectly delighted. Ottilie is a darling and will make Campbell a splendid wife. She is young, but that is a good fault, and she has extraordinary charm. A.G. [Grace] is worried a bit that she is inexperienced, but she really is capable and educatable. Last year when Grace was away, she was splendid and looked after the people and made everyone feel at home. I knew the minute Campbell came that he meant business. O. was a little frightened of him at first, but they soon became very chummy, and he lost no time. She was leaving on Saturday and warned by the tragic example of T.B.F. [Futcher] he sailed in bravely. They are extremely happy and are cooing like turtle doves. O. will stay on here tho Jared [Howard] wishes them both to go to Colonsay. Campbell does not wish to leave and I really think it would be best to stay quietly in this lovely spot. I have just got here. Ted and Muriel's [Eberts] cable came this a. m. to Oxford & was the first definite intimation I had, so I was in doubt whether it was Nona [Gwyn] or Ottilie until I got to the station. Ike & I discussed it as we came up and decided that either would do. I bet 100 to 1 on O. as no girl has a chance when she is about. All the boys this term have been devoted to her. Campbell is such a darling that I know she will adore him, and she will settle into a thoroughly good companion for him. . . ."

Ottilie and Campbell left Wales to visit her maternal cousins at a village near Glasgow during the final week of his stay in Britain. Low water in the Welsh streams made for poor fishing, so Revere turned his hand to sketching. Osler sent several of the pen and ink sketches to Campbell. Revere labelled these "Nona"; "Dad"; "Grandma" [Mrs. John Revere]; "Winchester Man" [profile] and "Front View"; "German Tourist"; and "Winchester College Man". Osler must have been delighted by his son's irreverant caricature of him. (Fig. 35).

Early in September, the Oslers returned to Oxford where Tom McCrae and Osler worked on a revision of the textbook for the 8th edition. Several proposed deadlines for its completion were missed, but W. O. finally turned over an acceptable draft to his junior colleague the following March. Tom and Amy (Gwyn) McCrae returned home on October 4 with her sister, Nona, and

Ottilie. Grace Osler had helped Ottilie select her trousseau in London while Osler showered presents on his "granddaughter-once-removed", including a beautiful watch for her birthday on September 20.

Campbell Howard and Ottilie Wright were married on December 27, 1911 in the bride's home, the city of Ottawa, Canada, among many friends of their families. After a short honeymoon, they reached Iowa for the reopening of classes early in January 1912. Osler's anticipation of the welcome the bride would receive in her new home was amusingly phrased. To Campbell he wrote: "Her things are perfectly lovely, and if Iowa City does not go wild over the bride of the P. of Med. I do not know the West." His observations when Ottilie was entertaining visitors at "The Open Arms" led Osler to assure Marjorie: "She has a good heart & is always so bright and cheery. She will be a great help with the students & doctors and she can talk most intelligently about nothing—which is a great art." Ottilie Howard was always able to welcome a stranger or put a shy guest at ease.

Osler's letters to Marjorie always included news of the progress of Revere, and affectionate wishes for Marjorie's two young boys. The baby, Thomas Bruce, was born on October 6, 1911. The Futchers selected Revere as one of Bruce's godfathers. Osler proudly mentioned that by the end of his holidays in January 1912 Revere had built a five foot liner with engines, which performed very successfully. He added, "I wish his head was as good as his hands and his heart, but he will be all right."[94]

Revere Osler suffered a severe attack of lobar pneumonia at Winchester College during March 1912, but the crisis passed favorably. With the textbook revision essentially completed, Osler and Grace were able to take Revere with them to convalesce for ten days in Northern Italy. His artistic sense was stimulated by the beautiful architecture in Venice. Osler sent Campbell a card on April 13, with a view of the University of Padua, and his greetings, "in which Realdo Colombo, Cesalpinus and Vesalius join." The next day Grace and Revere Osler returned to England. Osler attended the International Tuberculosis Congress in Rome from April 14–20. On his trip home, he stopped at Cannes on the French Riviera to see Dr. and Mrs. H. B. Jacobs. Doctor Jacobs recalled that Osler had "brought photos that Revere had taken in Venice —very remarkable for a boy, not of houses & boats, gondolas, etc. but details of capitals, friezes, gargoyles, etc.—little things which showed a rare power of observation and a fine artistic feeling". Osler was very proud of his son's photographs, and predicted Revere would become an architect or an artist.[95]

In his letter on April 28, 1912, to Marjorie Futcher, Osler mentioned Revere's full recovery, and his maturity, and also acknowledged the gift to Revere of a fine photograph of Bruce Futcher. He also made reference to W. S. Thayer's fortunate decision, for the Johns Hopkins faculty, students and his referred patients, in deciding to refuse a flattering offer from the Harvard Medical School. In the same letter, Osler expressed his excitement about Ottilie's pregnancy, and added the hope that a leading physician at McGill, such as C. F. Martin or H. A. Lafleur, would resign his professorship and open a place for Campbell. Osler had previously mentioned his protégé to Principal Peterson of the McGill University. In January, 1912, Grace Osler wrote the Principal about the new portrait of her husband at the Strathcona Medical Building. She added a postscript with the suggestion that available funds would now permit the recall of Campbell Howard to McGill.[96]

Campbell Howard brought Louis Baumann, Ph.D., from the Medical Chemical Laboratory at McGill, to Iowa with him so that he could start a similar research laboratory, and the new laboratory made useful contributions. Campbell Howard was elected an associate member of the Association of American Physicians in 1911, and the following year submitted his first paper to the program. He selected work conducted at Montreal with L. Baumann on "Metabolism of Scurvy in an Adult". Osler congratulated the authors in his letter of July 17, 1912, but regretted that the report had arrived too late for inclusion in the 1912 edition of the textbook. The study was performed on a 38-year-old male admitted in July, 1909, to Dr. H.A. Lafleur's service at the Montreal General Hospital. The literature review indicated that this was the first metabolic study performed on an adult with scurvy. Balance studies were done on a control diet before the addition of orange juice. More of the analyzed food constituents were retained after the addition of the fruit.[97]

Of interest in the correspondence at this time are references to the Oslers' August vacation in the Scottish Highlands. First they visited Tongue, in the far North, with Professor Somerville, and two young friends of Revere. They then spent a week at Skibo Castle with Andrew Carnegie. Revere caught trout despite much rain. The poor weather did not interfere greatly with the beautiful scenery, Osler's encounters with lay and professional friends or his examination of medical incunabula at the University of Edinburgh on the journey home.[98]

Campbell and Ottilie Howard's happiness about the birth, on November 4, 1912, of a boy destined to carry his grandfather's name was shared by "Docie O" and his family. His cable of congratulations was surely treasured by the parents, but has since been lost, and the only remaining expression of Osler's pleasure in the boy's birth is a letter to Marjorie. Revere Osler was naturally selected to be the boy's godfather. This continued the tradition in sequence. Osler was godfather to Campbell, and he in turn to Revere. William Osler gave an inscribed silver porringer to the young Palmer Howard.

In Osler's letter of December 10, 1912, to Marjorie, he also remarked: "It is nice to hear such good news of your Tom. Klebs the other day said he heard him give one of the best talks he ever listened to." Arnold Klebs began his friendship with Harvey Cushing in Baltimore. He also would see much of T. B. Futcher, who had shared the Franklin Street residence with H. B. Jacobs and Cushing. Klebs presumably continued his medical practice in Baltimore through the academic year, 1911–12, before he retired to Switzerland. He probably attended Futcher's talk on glycosuria before the Section on Genito-Urinary Diseases of the American Medical Association in Atlantic City on the morning of June 6, 1912. Harvey Cushing's paper, "The Internal Secretion of the Pituitary Body", presented to the combined sections of Surgery and Medicine, was delivered on the same day. Futcher included references to the experiments on the causes of glycosuria by Cushing's neurosurgical team.[99]

William Osler's whirlwind visit to America in 1913 included several highly significant occasions. He arrived in New York on April 13, visited Weir Mitchell and many Philadelphia friends the next day, and stayed at the Futchers' house from Tuesday, April 15 until Saturday, April 19, while the celebrations took place for the opening of the Henry Phipps Psychiatric Clinic at Johns Hopkins. His admirable opening address set the stage for the presentations of international leaders in psychiatry. He met old friends in small and large groups, including a dinner hosted by the Futchers on Friday evening.[100]

Osler secluded himself in the New Haven Graduates Club on April 19 to complete "A Way of Life" for reading the next evening to the Yale undergraduates. This inspirational address was reported in *The New York Times,* and published in several editions. A donor has arranged for its distribution annually to medical students at McGill University, and many share the belief that all students in medicine and the health professions today would profit from perusing its few pages.[101]

Osler also spoke with charm one evening at the Elizabethan Club of Yale on "Burton's Anatomy of Melancholy", as well as attending clinics every morning. The Silliman Lectures he presented in the afternoon provided an overview of medical history, with copious illustrations and biographical details full of insight and whimsy typical of his rare style. Delayed by Osler's other responsibilities and World War I, the task of publishing the lectures was finally accomplished in 1921 by Fielding H. Garrison.[102]

Osler spent April 29–30 in Boston and spoke at the opening ceremonies of the Peter Bent Brigham Hospital where "full-time" teachers would head the clinical departments. The introduction of this system at Johns Hopkins, and consideration of such reforms in medical education in London, were then absorbing much of his thought and writing. After renewing friendships and participating in meetings in New York, Philadelphia and Washington, Osler returned to stay overnight at the Futchers' house where Campbell and Ottilie Howard, with their baby, were also eager to exchange professional and personal news with the "Chief". On May 7 Osler gave the Johns Hopkins Nurses' commencement address in which he outlined the details of the seven virtues to which nurses should pay attention, "tact, tidiness, taciturnity, sympathy, gentleness, cheerfulness, all linked together by charity."[103] The following day Campbell presented a paper at the Association of American Physicians, and Osler travelled North to see old friends and relatives. His letter from Dundas, Ontario on May 9 to Marjorie thanked her for the hospitality and continued:

"I spent the morning with Gaylord at the laboratory [in Buffalo] & came on to Hamilton where Olmsted met me with his car & we came out here. I have seen all my old chums, and prowled about the scenes of my early wickedness. Nona [Gwyn] is looking stunning. The brother [Edmund Osler] is here from Winnipeg convalescing from an attack of pneumonia. I am off to Toronto tomorrow. Good-bye darling. 'Twas such a treat to see you & T.B. & those Futcher boys—to say nothing of old Campbell & his family."

From Toronto, Osler stopped off in Belleville to see Ned Milburn. He then attended the Medico-Chirurgical Society Meeting in

Montreal and renewed his contacts with his alma mater before embarking on May 15 for the comparative relaxation of a week at sea.

He reached Oxford on May 23, 1913, to find many professional obligations awaiting him, including the Oxford medical examinations, "The Open Arms" full of guests, and two patients of special importance. One was his beloved wife, whose wrists were stiff. The course of Grace Osler's arthralgia was not typical. Muirhead implied that she had borne minor ailments cheerfully, but that "she suffered especially from arthritis in her knee-joints". Margaret Revere recalls that she took "the cure" at Harrogate, and that she was advised to avoid eating those foods commonly prohibited following the diagnosis of gout.[104] The other patient, Edward Prince of Wales, came up to Magdalen College in 1912 and the Regius Professor received the request to oversee the Prince's health. The Prince participated actively in his college work and athletics. He suffered an attack of influenza in April, still had some symptoms and was underweight. He encountered a sympathetic counsellor in W.O. The call to military service in 1914 interrupted his attendance at Oxford but he sent Osler a framed photograph and silver inkstand as a souvenir. The inkstand was included with the silver willed by Lady Osler to her sister, Sue Chapin, who later gave it to the author while a student preparing to enter McGill College.[105]

Though Osler was increasingly involved with preparations for the XVIIth International Medical Congress, to take place in London in August, he still found some time for visitors and young people in Oxford and his personal correspondence. He wrote to Ottilie Howard on June 13, 1913. "Here are the girls—the darlings & Collis [Sands]. . . ." was on a card backed by a photograph of two Wright sisters and Susan and Margaret Revere (Fig. 34). In this card, and his August 1 letter to Marjorie, he mentioned the sorrow he shared with the surviving kin of Muriel Eberts. She had delivered her fifth child, Christopher, on May 5, 1913, but after a period of bed confinement with femoral phlebitis, she suffered an embolism and died suddenly on May 31.

By a strange coincidence, Ottilie Howard might have suffered the fate of her sister-in-law after the birth of her daughter, Muriel Marion, on November 16, 1913 in Iowa City. Early in the puerperium, Ottilie became gravely ill from puerperal sepsis with femoral-iliac thrombophlebitis. Probably pulmonary emboli further complicated the course. The baby was healthy at birth, but she was promptly weaned, lost weight for a few weeks, and then improved. T.B. and Marjorie Futcher both visited when Ottilie first became critically ill. Marjorie stayed a few weeks, and Ottilie's mother spent several months in Iowa City. Frequent cables and several letters with the Oslers were exchanged through March 1914 when Ottilie reached the convalescent stage, with residual chronic thrombophlebitis as a complication of the uterine infection. Though Osler's letter of February 1914 raised other diagnostic possibilities, it indicated his sympathy: "I do trust that all anxiety is now over. What a sad time the poor dear must have had, and you must have been wild with apprehension. I dare say now she will make a rapid recovery. Thanks for your cables. We have been so worried. I know how risky these pneumococci infections are— or was it entirely a post-appendicular affair? You must have found it very hard to do your work with such a load at your heart. I saw J. [Jared] and Maggie [Howard] the other day. They are at Grosvenor Square, settling everything. Marjorie must have been a comfort & Tom [Futcher]. I hope the baby is thriving."

Campbell's sister-in-law, Margaret Howard, became Lady Strathcona and Mount Royal upon the death of her father on January 21, 1914. He had been a very generous benefactor to the McGill Medical College and University, the International Association of Medical Museums and many other educational programs in Canada and Britain. Osler may have made suggestions for the memorial tribute in the *Lancet.* [106]

The Osler family had spent a happy time together in Oxford. In Osler's letter to Marjorie, written just after Christmas, he regretted her absence and wished she could have seen Revere. "He has taken to etching & today finished his first bit. He is deeply interested in art & becoming so well read in literature." Revere may have begun etching during the April, 1912, trip to Italy. His renewed interest in art and literature was mentioned in Osler's letters to H. B. Jacobs in December, 1913, and to J. William White in the following month. [107]

In another letter to Marjorie about January 15, 1914, he referred to Ottilie's illness, their own Christmas activities and the improvement in Grace's wrists. He also mentioned his satisfaction with Mr. Enoch, a new librarian-secretary, and also the "circus at the Hopkins". The service of Miss B.O. Humpton, Osler's former secretary at the Hopkins, had been excellent, and he had had difficulty finding a suitable replacement in Oxford. Apart from Revere's governess-turned-secretary, Nicola Smith, others had not been satisfactory. From this reference it appears that Mr. Enoch began work in January, 1914. Osler's account book included the secretary's salary in June, 1914, and the "Autobiographical Notes" mentioned that Mr. Enoch left for War Service during June, 1915.[108]

In the January letter to Marjorie, Osler elaborated on the Hopkins situation: "I am so grieved for Barker. I hope Thayer will be able to take it as to bring in a young outsider—unless C. [possibly Campbell]—would raise the devil." Though covered fully elsewhere it seems appropriate to outline here what was taking place at the Johns Hopkins Institutions in 1914, and continue the story of the Department of Medicine during Osler's lifetime.

The Johns Hopkins Medical School and Hospital were in the midst of introducing the full-time system for the clinical faculty. Osler's longtime colleague, Professor William H. Welch, had favored this reorganization, and introduced the idea to the Rockefeller's General Education Board. Osler kept himself informed, and in general favored the original system of allowing consultation privileges to the clinicians. His successor, as Chairman of the Department of Medicine, Professor Lewellys F. Barker, deliberated carefully, but on January 17, 1914, he reported to the Hospital Board that he could not give up consultation practice as the Surgeon-in-Chief, W. S. Halsted, and Pediatrician-in-Chief, John Howland, had agreed to do. The position in medicine was immediately offered to W. S. Thayer, who also declined. In the spring, Theodore C. Janeway of Columbia University, New York, was appointed Professor of Medicine and Physician-in-Chief to the hospital, effective July 1, 1914. Doctors Barker and Thayer continued as part-time clinical teachers.

The task of reorganizing the Department of Medicine was complicated by increasing involvement in military responsibilities for all the full-time and clinical staff. At the age of forty-five, after a little over three years as chairman, Dr. Janeway announced his intention to resign and return to New York; unfortunately, however, he died in Baltimore on December 27, 1917. Dr. Thayer indicated he would accept the position after completing his military duties. He held the chair from 1919 until the spring of 1921, when he resigned. He continued, however, as Clinical Professor of Medicine until his death in 1932.[109]

Osler predicted Ottilie's rapid recovery in his March 12, 1914, letter to Campbell, and also complimented him on the publication of his paper on bronchiectasis. Campbell had presented this paper in May, 1913, to the Association of American Physicians in Atlantic

City after studying four patients in the University of Iowa Hospital. Osler commented: "It seems to me that the disease has increased very much of late. I have seen a good many cases over here and at present have a remarkable one under observation which has lasted some 15 years."[110]

World War I, which had been brewing between the Central European Powers and the Western European Allies and Russia for several years, finally broke out in 1914. The entry of the United States during 1917 turned a stalemate into the Allied Victory in November 1918. A brief review of the effects of the War on Sir William Osler and the Howard family will facilitate an understanding of the events covered in the Osler correspondence.

CHAPTER V

Stresses of World War I

ON AUGUST 4, 1914 a sudden and devastating change occurred in the social and professional lives of many persons in Europe and the British Commonwealth, including the Oslers. For nine years, while keeping a devoted watch over Revere's growth and education, the parents had participated in the British medical, academic, and related social life. Despite the smoldering tensions in central Europe, Lady Osler and Revere had sailed for Canada and the United States in advance of Osler. When the bombardments of World War I broke out, they immediately returned to Britain.

Revere's successful matriculation to enter Oxford University in the autumn had brought his father's aspirations for him close to realization. With the outbreak of war, Revere accepted the advice to pursue his studies for the term while he entered the officers' training corps. Most students at Oxford were replaced by families of European refugees, and some University buildings were turned into hospitals.

Osler's medical student classes were suspended, but he added a heavy schedule of duties as consultant to the civilian health authorities and Honorary Colonel in the British Army. He acted unofficially as a consultant also for the Canadian Army Medical Corps, and paid frequent visits to North American hospitals, which were supported by the Red Cross and other private groups. After 1917, he played the same role for the medical components of the American Expeditionary Force. To the sick and wounded, the medical personnel and the families of each of them, Osler was a trusted medical advisor. He fully earned the affectionate sobriquet of "Consoler-General".

The gracious hospitality of Grace Osler at "The Open Arms"

played a large role in relieving the stresses, and comforting the griefs, of the War for many Canadian and American visitors. Without Grace, Osler's part could not have been fully carried out. On short notice, individuals or large groups were welcomed to England, and dispatched abroad. The wounded Rhodes Scholar, Wilder Penfield, was among many North Americans who convalesced at the Osler home. The tribute of a senior officer in the American Army expressed the widely felt gratitude.[111]

Osler was a leading contributor to national studies on the unusual manifestations of fevers, nephritis, disordered action of the heart and nervous symptoms among the soldiers at the front. He participated vigorously in campaigns to control the spread of tuberculosis and venereal diseases among soldiers, and also the civilian population.

The rising toll of war casualties, and his concern about disputes in military medical administration, apparently contributed to symptoms of mental depression, which Osler could not always disguise by continuing his heavy professional and social activities. While wholeheartedly supporting the allied military effort, Osler urged restraint in the bitterness of the British public and press towards enemy citizens. When peace came, he quickly joined movements to send food and supplies to the destitute in war-torn countries.

Most families of the Western European allies, and of the opposing countries, lost men in battle, and some were decimated by the immediate ravages of war or the accompanying disease and famine. Deaths in battle took young men from the Osler, Howard, Wright families, and those of cousins, friends and associates in all spheres of their lives. Though duty at the front or sea was dangerous for medical personnel, service at base hospitals was relatively safe.

Thomas McCrae, T.B. Futcher and Campbell Howard were among many British subjects living in the United States who served with the Canadian expeditionary force. Thomas McCrae, a Canadian graduate residing in Philadelphia, took leave from his professorial duties at Jefferson Medical College. He travelled to Britain as a private citizen, enlisted in the Canadian army and was in charge of the medical wards of the Ontario Military Hospital at Orpington, Kent, near London. He served as Lieutenant Colonel from June 25, 1917 until he resigned from duty on September 30 of the same year. Thomas B. Futcher, also a University of Toronto medical graduate, left his consulting practice and position as Associate Professor of Clinical Medicine at John Hopkins in September, 1917, with the purpose of replacing T. McCrae. Futcher was commissioned on September 12, 1917 in England, and was immediately posted as Lieutenant-Colonel to No. 16 Canadian (Ontario) General Hospital at Orpington. He resigned his commission on April 1, 1918, in England.[112]

During the war, letters from the Oslers to the Howard and Futcher families were sporadic and usually brief. Some, however, were filled with vivid descriptions or poignant expressions of sorrow, and added important details to the Osler-Howard story.

Osler's letter written about October 10, 1914, to Marjorie began with his regrets that he had been cheated from visiting the Futchers. After war had been declared in August 1914, Osler had been forced to cancel plans to attend the celebration for the 25th year of the Johns Hopkins Hospital in Baltimore. Osler mailed his message "Looking Back" for W. S. Thayer to read on October 5. He referred to the teaching of the medical student in the hospital as "a method initiated in Holland, developed in Edinburgh, matured in London, and long struggled for here, but never attained until the Johns Hopkins Medical School was started".[113]

His letter to Marjorie continued about the refugee professors and their wives from Louvain University, who now occupied a large part of "The Open Arms." In Osler's words: "You should see the Gallerie Lafayette in the drawing-room—full of Belgian Professors wives. Such clothing and making over! And they all have bustles, inside & out! We have sixteen families now—nearly 100 & I fear it will be a long job. Fortunately the Professors in the Science depts can be helped by the Rockefeller funds. I wish you could see my upstairs library—in the blue room—very busy place now. Muz [Grace] writes in one corner. I dig at books on the table & Ike Walton is sketching a book plate. He is deep in English literature & art. He has been in the [Officer's] Training Corps, but does not take very kindly to the work. He will continue next term & apply for a commission when ready. He wanted to go off to India with one of the Territorial regiments in which a chum got a billet, but the Col. of the O.T.C. said he was not fit.[114] We are all very hopeful—& the country is coming forward splendidly. There are thousands of recruits here & the Schools is a base Hospital! . . ."

The unusual crowding of the family must have disturbed Osler's writing. The national surge of defiance against the German powers was highly emotional, and put pressure on all young men to volunteer for combat service. Revere was not well-developed in physique, but his father was probably more important than the Colonel of the Officers' Training Corps in influencing him to remain at Oxford University. Osler's last remark reflected the changed environment of Oxford. The Examination Schools building of the University housed the 1,000 beds and operating rooms of the 3rd Southern General Hospital. The Radcliffe Infirmary and other components of the University were also used for military activities. Many of the staff of the Infirmary were commissioned to serve in these units while they continued their usual civilian duties.[115]

Much had happened before the events mentioned in Osler's letter of April 23, 1915, to Marjorie. No. 3 Canadian General Hospital was mobilized, with the medical staff provided by McGill University. Colonel Birkett, the Dean of the Medical College, assumed command of the Unit. W.W. Francis had recovered his health sufficiently to be appointed on the medical staff. Campbell Howard had received a leave of absence from Iowa University on February 21, 1915. He joined this hospital as a Major. After preliminary training at Valcartier camp near Quebec, No. 3 Canadian General Hospital reached England in May, 1915.

Revere did not return to Oxford for the winter term. His interests had been literary and his physical talents did not give an indication of martial combat. Presumably through respect and friendship for his father, Colonel Birkett offered Revere the post of assistant quartermaster with the rank of 2nd Lieutenant. He joined the advance party of the McGill Unit at Cliveden (Taplow) in February, 1915. When the full complement was encamped beside the Beechborough Park Hospital at Shorncliffe, Kent, in May, Revere received further training for the duties which he would perform in a 1200 bed military hospital.[116]

The newly arrived Canadians had only a few weeks to meet old friends, for example the Osler and Wright families in Oxford. No. 3 Canadian General Hospital reached France on June 17, 1915 and set up in tents at Camiers, about twelve miles south of Boulogne. Lieutenant Colonel John McCrae, who had written "In Flanders Fields" during his duty in the trenches at the defense of Ypres, took charge of the medical service. The admission of patients did not occur until the second half of August, and only the quartermaster and his assistant escaped the general boredom. In Osler's words, to Marjorie Futcher: "Poor old C. [Campbell] has had a weary wait! It is too bad. They only open, we hear, on Aug. 1st. [actually later] There have been no patients lately. Revere writes very amusing letters, but they have evidently had a trying time."[117]

A report on patients that Campbell Howard had studied at the University of Iowa appeared in a recent issue of the *Johns Hopkins Hospital Bulletin.* This received a favorable review in the *Lancet,* probably due to Osler's suggestion, if not from his pen. On August 14, 1915, he encouraged Campbell's professional interests with the following words: "Very good account of your Mediastinitis paper in Lancet of this week. I hope you have cases at last. Look out for the nephritis which is most interesting. I saw 8 cases yesterday at Paignton." As a volunteer consultant since its organization in 1914, Osler paid regular visits to the American Women's War Hospital at Paignton. The form of nephritis which occurred in the conditions of trench warfare was later the subject of conferences in which Osler participated. His report was based on 113 soldiers admitted to the Canadian Hospital at Taplow, thirty to the American Hospital in Paignton and others at the hospitals in Oxford.[118]

Late in August, 1915, the surgeon J. B. Murphy offered Campbell Howard the position of Head of the Medical Service at Mercy Hospital in Chicago. Murphy had probably met him through Dr. Charles J. Rowan, an assistant of his from 1902–06, who had been appointed the Professor and Head of the Department of Surgery at Iowa in January, 1914. Murphy became Chief of the Surgical Service at Mercy Hospital, and Professor of Surgery, Northwestern University Medical School in 1908. Campbell's godfather and beloved "Chief" was guarded in his endorsement of Murphy's offer, preferring that Campbell would relocate eventually at one of the Montreal hospitals associated with McGill University: "That is a very flattering offer (you did not enclose the letter) but of course you must have the details you ask for. There are two points in my mind—first if not academic I would hesitate, & second, I do not like J. B. [Murphy of Chicago] personally. Perhaps that is because I do not know him well. He is a big surgeon but how he is as a man & colleague I do not know. Men who do know him say his exterior is the only thing agin him.[119] I hope to cross on Wednesday [September 8] & we can talk it over. I should like to see you back in Montreal with a good clinic at one of the Hospitals. The school needs you. I had hoped to talk with [Principal] Peterson this summer about it but he has not come over."

Campbell declined Murphy's proposals. Osler's letter of September 6 also mentioned Revere's unrest at continued service behind the battle lines and the probability that Campbell's family might soon arrive in Oxford: "Revere is worrying about whether his job is the right one or not. He feels that he is not earning his salt. I suppose he has not got into the work at wh. I dare say he is an awful duffer. Grace hears that they [Mrs. H. P. Wright, three daughters and Hilda] sail on the 6th. I hope you will be able to get a week's leave. It will be delightful to have them all here. I am looking forward to a winter of great pleasure with the kiddies."

Osler's projected visit to No. 3 Canadian General Hospital in France took place between September 8 and 15. His thorough inspection allowed ample time for conversations with Revere, Bill Francis, Col. Birkett, Campbell and Jack McCrae. With official approval, and under McCrae's guidance, Osler also visited units within the battle zone, and another British hospital near the coast where the typhoid and paratyphoid cases of the district were concentrated. They were remarkably few, in his opinion, for the large size of the expeditionary force.

Revere's post as assistant quartermaster was obviously not haz-ardous, but the Canadian medical officers expressed their pleasure with his work. Osler never mentioned that he was uncomfortable about his son's protected position, or his fears that Revere might chose to serve with the combatant forces. After they met in France, however, he must have understood that Revere's con-science was troubling him, as his wife was well aware. He also confirmed the recent arrival at Oxford of Ottilie Howard, her two children and her mother in his September 17, 1915, letter to Camp-bell:

"Ottilie & Grace met me at the station. O. looks so well—not a bit changed. The children are splendid & the house will be very satisfactory. I do hope you will be able to come soon. I told O. that it might be some time as there was a new regulation as to leave. It was such a pleasure to see you all, & the outlook for work seems satisfactory. Let me know about literature at any time. Revere has decided to sit tight for a time, but it is only natural that he should feel restive. I do not believe he has enough to do—& that is very hard for him."[120]

Campbell Howard obtained leave to visit his family in Oxford early in November, but before Muriel's second birthday, on the 16th, he returned to his unit. A response was required to a recent letter from the University of Iowa. A review of the background and the developments since he had left Iowa City will clarify the actions covered in the correspondence of Osler and Howard at this time.

Although the United States had not yet entered World War I, several large medical schools had staffed volunteer units to serve abroad with the Allied forces. The doctors usually spent one year in rotation. Campbell understood that President Macbride would recommend an indefinite leave of absence for him from duties at the University of Iowa in February, 1915. At the next meeting of the Finance Committee of the State Board of Education, Doctor Howard's leave of absence was authorized, but his proposals for the reorganization, staffing and salaries in the Department of Theory and Practice of Medicine were approved "with the understanding that this arrangement is in force until July 1, 1915, only." At the end of August, 1915, the Dean of the Medical College, L.W. Dean, considered that the work in this Department was not being carried out satisfactorily. A recent letter (not extant) from Howard did not assure his early return to Iowa. The teaching and patient load at the University was increasing. In view of the extreme importance of this department to the College of Medicine, the Dean advised that a permanent head for the Department of Theory and Practice of Medicine be secured as soon as a competent man could be found. The Dean's recommendation was approved at the August 31, 1915 meeting of the State Board of Education, under Chairman D. D. Murphy. A copy has not been located of the letter written by the Dean during September, 1915 to Campbell Howard, but he interpreted its import that he must return to the University of Iowa before the second semester began in February, 1916, or else resign from the University.

Osler believed that Campbell would serve the Allied cause more effectively in a civilian capacity than in a military hospital, and that it was not proper to let him sacrifice his academic future. McGill University had undertaken to supply the medical officers for No. 3 Canadian General Hospital. Osler wrote Principal W. Peterson on November 15, 1915 to initiate procedures through the Canadian Department of Militia to relieve Campbell from service. At this time, Osler also had reached the conclusion that McGill should found a modern clinic for research and teaching, so he included the suggestion that Campbell now be offered a senior faculty appointment at McGill in this letter:

"Campbell Howard has had word from his University to return for the Spring term if he wishes to retain his post. Gen. Carleton Jones is grumbling a bit at this, but it would not be fair to keep him longer. After all he will have given a year & it would not do to get out of the line of academic work. He has just turned down a most flattering offer from Chicago chiefly on account of the man who made it—not a very satisfactory colleague. I wish we could see him back at McGill. An investigator of his type is needed with advanced clinical methods. Do you think there is any possibility?"[121]

Campbell Howard had received Colonel Birkett's approval to approach the Director General of the Medical Services of the Canadian Expeditionary Force. Surgeon-General Jones, however, told him that he should make his request to be relieved from duty through McGill University. Campbell wrote Principal Peterson on November 15. The Principal had also received the letter from Osler, and one from Colonel Birkett, before November 30 when he wrote General Sir Sam Hughes, the Canadian Minister of Militia. The Principal informed Campbell Howard about his action and remarked: "I think you are quite right in preparing to resume work at Iowa, and only wish we had a fine post here for you to tumble into instead of going there." After receiving General Hughes prompt reply Principal Peterson informed Osler on December 6, 1915:

"I wrote at once to the Minister [Hughes] about Campbell Howard and have his reply stating that he has forwarded a copy of my letter to General Carson in London asking him to look into the matter.

"I have written to General Carson begging that he will give it personal attention, and expressing the hope that he has power to deal with it. I suggest that you find out from Carson what he is doing in regard to the matter, and if there is any delay, send me a cable when I shall take it up again directly with the Minister at Ottawa.

"I fear there are no appointments [for Campbell Howard] here at present, but shall remember what you say.

"All my friends were delighted with your kind and generous subscription to the [University] Magazine. The December number is just out, and I hope you will like it when you get your copy."[122]

Osler mentioned his correspondence with Principal Peterson and recent family news in his letters to Campbell on November 18 and December 17, 1915. He also expressed regrets about the severe attack of pneumonia suffered by Lieutenant Colonel Yates, Admistrative Officer at the McGill unit, and remarked: "I hope you will move soon. I felt sure that was an impossible hole for winter." Osler had formed this opinion about the Camiers camp during his September visit, but expressed himself publicly only after the announcement that its location would be changed. Late in December General John Carson, the senior Canadian officer in London, issued the orders to recall Campbell Howard from France. Ottilie left the children in Oxford and returned to Canada with her husband on a troopship. On January 29, 1916, he was placed on the inactive list of the Canadian Army Medical Corps.

Osler believed that his protégé should move on from Iowa. At about Campbell's age, Osler's own career had included transfers to Pennsylvania, and soon again to Johns Hopkins. Thomas A. Warthin recently permitted the use of a letter from Osler to his father, Dr. Alfred S. Warthin, Professor of Pathology at the University of Michigan. When Osler learned that the chair of medicine was vacant on January 15, 1916, he sent Professor Warthin a strong recommendation about Campbell Howard, "a good teacher, an ideal worker and a fine character with a powerful and unusual influence on young men . . . he has done splendidly [in Iowa]." However, T. A. Warthin has discovered that the delivery of Osler's letter was delayed by wartime hazards until after the Committee at Michigan had made its report.

The warmth of Campbell Howard's welcome early in February by his colleagues at Iowa would probably have kept him from transferring at that time. His description of the medical and surgical problems of modern warfare and their management was printed in the University newspaper, and he responded to demands for lectures on related topics before medical and lay groups throughout World War I.[123]

Professor Howard was absent when new rules governing the clinical work were adopted at the June 7, 1915, meeting of the faculty of the College of Medicine. The new Department of Pediatrics was given the responsibility for children up to twelve years of age, and also for patients of any age admitted to the Hospital with the common contagious diseases. After Campbell Howard's return from overseas, this rule was altered. Effective February 1, 1916, all patients thirteen years of age or older in the University Hospital had to be under the care of the Department of Medicine. Appointments to clinical duties, laboratory services and research also were made with the approval of the reinstated Professor of Medicine. In 1915, the number of admissions of children and adults to the hospital was greater. It was likely to increase further as a consequence of the passage of the Perkins Bill by the Iowa State Legislature. This bill provided for the medical care of poor children. Dr. Graham of Des Moines was secured to be superintendent of the University Hospital effective January 1, 1916.[124]

Osler's note of February 4, 1916 to Ottilie Howard gave news of her children whom he often visited during the tea hour at their grandmother's house. Although both welcomed him, the imaginative spirit of this "grown-up" drew especially demonstrative responses from Muriel, as it did from Susan Revere Baker and other little girls. In his words:

"Anything sweeter than your lassie [Muriel] was never seen—a perfect picture, such cheeks and as merry as her *MA*. She rushes out to meet me at the top of the stairs every evening. She grows bonnier every day. Old Pom-Pom [Palmer] is A.1. but he does not pay much attention to me if others are about. . . ."

The children still remember many activities in the company of Revere and family members during their stay in Oxford, but their playful encounters with the Osler men ended during May, 1916.[125] (Fig. 42)

The fighting at the front became more intense in 1916. Revere continued to be dissatisfied with the shelterd life of assistant quartermaster at a base hospital, while the wounded were coming in and his friends were on active service. After some delay, Revere was released from the Canadian Army Medical Corps and returned to Oxford on March 6. On the following day, he filed his application to transfer to the British Artillery. More than a year's military service had also added physical maturity to the young man, now twenty years of age. On March 8, Osler wrote Marjorie Futcher:

"When are we to see you again? This horrid war may last another two years. Revere got home on 6th to arrange his transfer to the Imperial Army. He feels he should be in the fighting line, and hopes to join the artillery. He is in A.1. form, hard as nails, and long association with Jack McCrae has made him a bit bloodthirsty."

During the few days at home, Revere and his father spent much time together. His father wrote an old friend: "He has got his line in life—perfectly devoted to literature & to books—a great comfort to me . . ." Like many other parents, however, they steeled themselves for the worst. Grace Osler confessed to another: "I suppose our turn will come."[126]

During 1916, Osler suffered emotional strain with periods of mental depression and loss of weight. Revere completed training as an Artillery Officer in England and joined his battery during October at the front near the Ancre and Somme Rivers. In his November 2, 1916, letter to Marjorie Futcher, Osler recollected the death in action of young Harry Howard at Ypres on May 9, 1915, and mentioned a recent wound of Arthur Howard. Although he revealed his fears about Revere to his former associate, W. S. Thayer, he usually suppressed his apprehension and wrote proudly about Revere's service, as to Marjorie: "Revere is off and writes such cheery letters from the Somme district. He is in the Ammunition column at present & deep in mud & driving mules. We must copy some of his letters & send them about. He has developed so much—you would hardly know him."[127]

Osler was also upset by troubles in the administration of the Canadian Expeditionary Force. From his visits to the Canadian Army Hospitals, he had formed a favorable opinion of Surgeon-General Guy Carleton Jones. Osler was incensed by the manner in which the Canadian Minister of Militia, General Sir Sam Hughes, ordered that the sick and wounded Canadian troops be segregated into Canadian convalescent hospitals without clearing this order with the British Army authorities or General Jones. Hughes then appointed a commission of inquiry, composed of political partisans, who prepared a damaging report. This resulted in the recall of General Jones. Osler resigned as consultant to the Canadian Army Hospitals in October, 1916. Within two months, Hughes left the Cabinet. Prime Minister Sir Robert Borden replaced him with Sir George Perley, and Major General Richard E. W. Turner assumed command of the Canadian Expeditionary Force. Early in 1917, the report of a second board of inquiry was followed by the reinstatement of General Jones, after which Osler withdrew his resignation.[128]

During the autumn of 1916, before the United States declared war, the situation of the Allies grew serious, and Campbell Howard wrote Osler for advice regarding further military service in England or France. Many febrile illnesses afflicted the soldiers in proximity to the trench warfare. The typhoid group could be readily recognized by bacteriological tests, and the louse-transmitted typhus fever was rarely encountered in France. A new incapacitating but non-fatal illness, Trench fever, was diagnosed, however, by its characteristic symptoms and course, which distinguished it from other "fevers of unknown origin". After a short period of fever and weakness, many suffered severe pains in the shins, less often in the knees, hips, or calf muscles. Other symptoms and signs resembled a mild form of typhus fever. Later it was found that transmission might occur from the crushed bodies or excrements of lice into scarified skin, and evidence accumulated

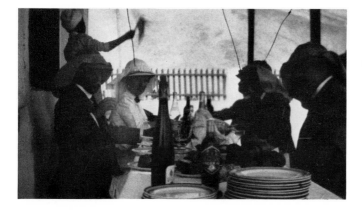

27.   Letter from Wm. Osler to C.P. Howard in
Iowa City, mailed September 7, 1910

28.   Aboard the *S.S. Seti* on the Nile,
February-March 1911

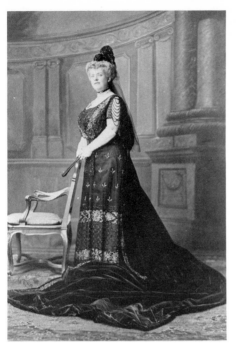

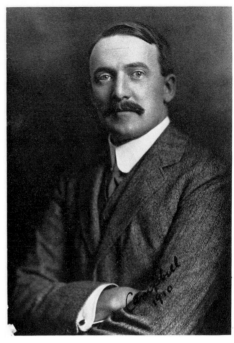

29. Lady Osler presented at
Court, June 1911

30. Campbell Howard, 1910

32. Ottilie Wright presented
at Court during ceremonies preceding
coronation of King George V

31. Ottilie Wright, Oxford(?), 1911

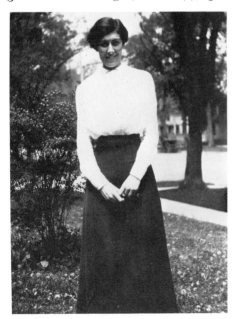

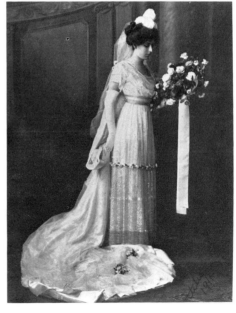

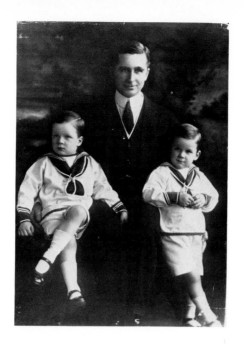

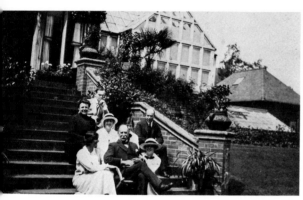

33. (left to right) Palmer Howard Futcher, Thomas Barnes Futcher, M.D., T. Bruce Futcher, c. 1914

34. At *The Open Arms*, June 1913

35. Revere's amusing drawings of Nona Gwyn, his father, "grandma," and a fellow "Winchester Man"

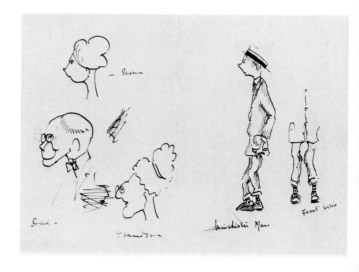

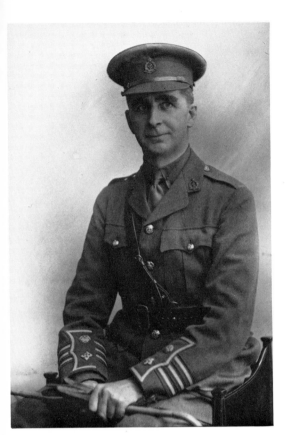

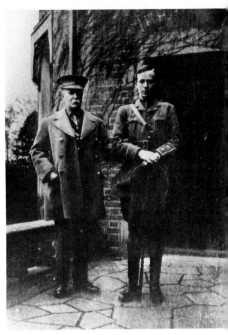

36. Lieutenant-Colonel T.B. Futcher, C.A.M.C., 1917

37. "The Colonel and the Lieutenant (Revere Osler)," 1915

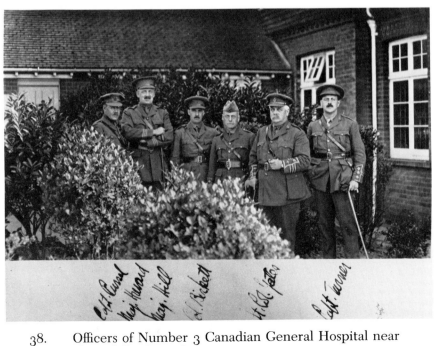

38. Officers of Number 3 Canadian General Hospital near Shorncliffe, Kent, June 1915

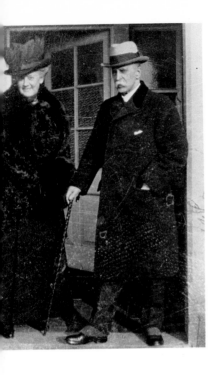

39. Sir William and Lady Osler, Oxford, c. 1917
40. Campbell, Muriel, and Palmer Howard, Iowa City, c. 1917
41. Lady Osler with Muriel and Palmer Howard at a summer cottage, Southbourne-on-Sea, Hants, August 1920
42. Hunting Easter eggs at 13 Norham Gardens, April 23, 1916

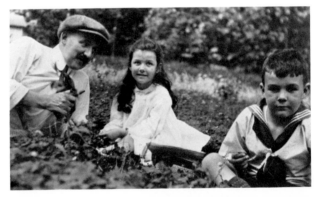

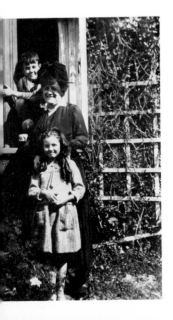

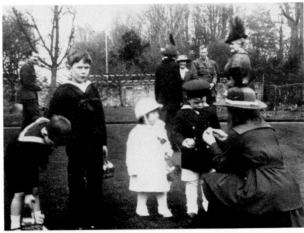

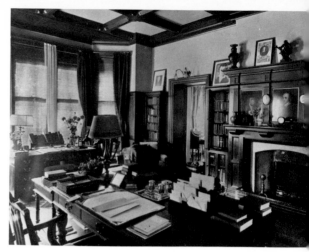

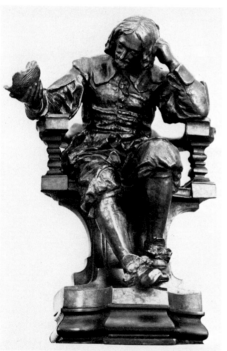

43. Library at 13 Norham Garden
during preparation of
Bibliotheca Osleriana,
photograph by Dr. John
Fulton

44. Osler's replica of H. Pegram's
statue of Sir Thomas Browne
at Norwich

45. Large oak table used as desk
by Sir William Osler at Oxford

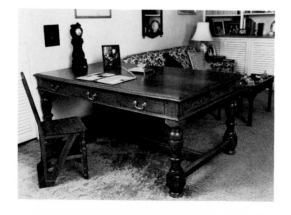

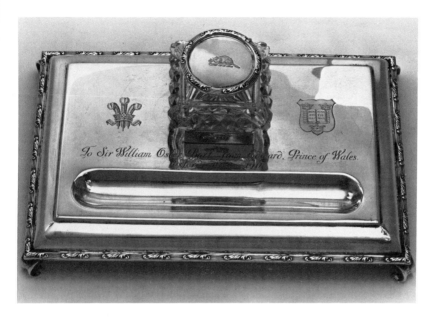

46–47   Silver inkstand engraved: "To Sir William Osler,
         Bart. from Edward, Prince of Wales, Oxford,
         1912–1914."

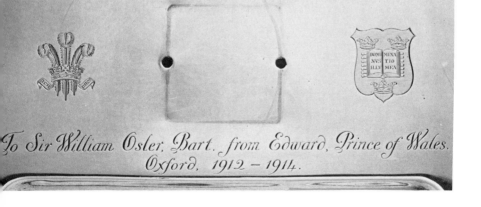

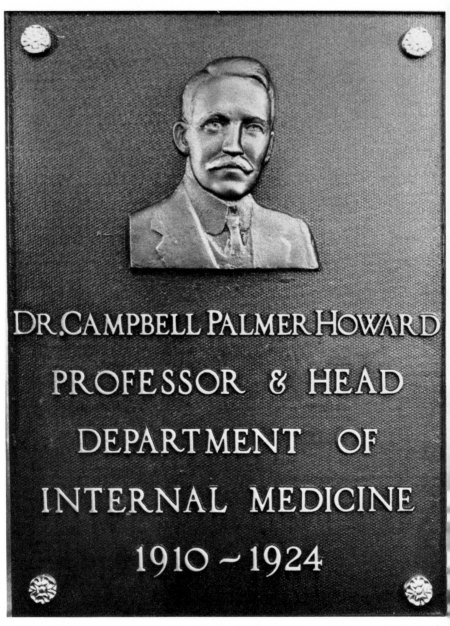

DR. CAMPBELL PALMER HOWARD

PROFESSOR & HEAD

DEPARTMENT OF

INTERNAL MEDICINE

1910 ~ 1924

48.   Plaque erected by the Medical Alumni Association and situated in the Department of Internal Medicine, University of Iowa, Iowa City

that the causative agent resembled, but was not identical to, that of typhus. Osler was greatly interested in the clarification of this disease. He helped Major Strong publish, and then he reviewed the report.[129]

In his letter to Campbell on December 4, 1916, Osler responded to Campbell's offer, reviewed the current medical situation and touched on family matters:

"I am much touched by your kind offer. Let matters rest until the spring & then if I can hear of a good medical billet for the summer I will cable or write. You are still I suppose officially attached to the C.A.M.C. The shortage of men in France is beginning to tell & very many are laid up. This P.U.O. [pyrexia or fever of unknown origin] is knocking out a good number of medical men. Norman Gwyn has had 3 weeks of it. Archie Malloch is down. No typhoid or paratyphoid reactions & it seems longer than the Trench fever; tho it may have the curious pains [in] shins & feet as a sequel.

"Ike is in the thick of it at last—went over 2 mos ago to the Battery A. 59th Division & has been in all this Ancre push. He writes very cheerfully and is with such nice men. He says he is happier than at any time since the war began.

"We are all rejoicing in the exit of Sam Hughes. He treated [G.C.] Jones disgracefully. A committee has been appointed to review the Bruce [Canadian Medical] report. Borden asked me to join but I did not care to be mixed up in it. To have put Turner in command here is splendid. He is a soldier.

"Mrs. Wright & Marion & Billie come to us for Xmas. Harry [Wright] seems doing such good work. I enclose a letter to my darling [Muriel]. Love to Ottilie.

Yours ever, Docie. O."

Osler mentioned to Marjorie the general satisfaction that Lloyd George was "at the helm". Despite the advice of his friends, and the urging of his wife to slow down after spending ten days in bed with bronchopneumonia after Christmas, he worked himself at his usual driving pace. Revere was involved in heavy action at the front for several months. Osler had consulted Campbell's former Commanding Officer before writing both the Howards on March 1, 1917. In the letter to Ottilie he mentioned how much he missed her children, and anticipated Revere's leave. He concluded: "We are doing well on our rations—& the belts not yet tightened." To Campbell he wrote:

"I had a chat with [Col. H.S.] Birkett two days ago & he thinks it would not be fair to ask you to give up the chair to come over —tho. he should like so much to have you back. The possibility of war will make a difference, as units no doubt will be asked for. I do not suppose it will make any difference about your citizenship. We are very much excited about the situation in the U.S. and the two Boston women [Grace and her sister Sue] are wild with excitement.

"I am all right again, but am trying to be a bit less rushed. Nothing very special. Same run of nervous cases & P.U.O.'s, less nephritis. The Heart Hospital work is interesting. Colin [Russel] & [J.C.] Meakins are both there. How lucky you did not go to [J.B.] Murphy! Poor fellow! another angina from an over-driven machine. Arthur Howard has had another flesh wound—doing well. I saw J & M [Jared & Maggie Howard] last week."

William Osler, Clifford Allbutt and James MacKenzie collaborated in the organization of the British Army Heart Hospital at Hampstead, Surrey, in 1916. Thomas Lewis, J. Parkinson and John C. Meakins, later Professor of Medicine at McGill, were in charge of services there. Colin K. Russel of McGill was also on the Heart Hospital staff. Osler visited the hospital every week until 1918 when it was moved to Colchester, Essex.[(130)]

His letter to Marjorie on March 9, 1917, contained similar news about Arthur Howard's second wound on February 14, and Revere's battle experiences. Marjorie was pregnant, and answered Osler's hopes for a girl when Gwendolen was born on July 16, 1917. The United States had declared war against Germany on April 16. Many of Osler's kin folk and friends had lost sons in battle, including Campbell Gwyn on April 9, 1917, and William R. Wright on May 13, 1917. Osler and his wife masked their apprehension by long hours of work related to the war effort. Osler also sought relief from the grim concerns of the present by spending absorbing hours of reflexion among his treasured books, and frequently successful searches to fill open spaces in his plan of the Bibliotheca.

Near the end of May, 1917, Revere obtained leave. His father noted: "he went away a boy and returned a hardened man". For ten happy days, to the great delight of his father, Revere divided his time between fishing for trout and collecting classical books.[(131)]

Revere's dangerous assignment at the front was very much a preoccupation for his parents. Some of the Oslers' close friends stationed near the front were aware of the identity and location of Revere's battery. Harvey Cushing was among them and by chance he was quite near the British Casualty Clearing Station where the gravely wounded Revere was taken on the evening of

August 29, 1917. A direct hit from a shell had killed or wounded nine out of the twenty men and officers while preparing to move forward the guns in their battery. Harvey Cushing reached Revere to find him conscious, but with shrapnel wounds penetrating his chest and abdomen. Major George W. Crile, the famous surgeon and a pioneer expert in blood replacement, helped William Darrach perform emergency surgery that night, but Revere did not live to see the dawn break over a Flanders field. He was laid under the Union Jack while American army medical officers and his father's friends were among those who heard the "Last Post". Later that afternoon Harvey Cushing's telegram reached his mother and father that he had been gravely wounded. At 9 p.m. a telephone call from the War Office informed them of his death. "We are heart broken, but thankful to have the precious memory of his loving life."[132]

The consolation and support William and Grace Osler gave each other can hardly be comprehended. Osler immediately began to write many others he loved. To Marjorie Futcher his words included: "Poor Grace! I am desolated for her sake more than for my own. She did so much for him and was such a good influence. . . . It was too much to expect that he would escape. The wonder he has been spared so long. . . ." Osler regarded Marjorie, Campbell and Ottilie and certain other long-known friends to be "his children", and he carried this affectionate feeling on to his children's children. To clarify small mistakes and to fill a line omitted in Cushing's biography, Osler's letter of August 31, 1917, to Campbell and Ottilie Howard follows:

"You will be desolated, as we are, at the loss of the dear boy. We have been steeling our hearts for the blow, but now that it has come the bitterness is much more than we thought. Dear laddie! he loathed the whole business of war, and I dare say is glad to be at peace out of the hell of the past six months. Was it not a blessing that Harvey [Cushing] was with him? This really softens the blow. We have had no details so far. Harvey wired yesterday dangerously wounded but "conscious & comfortable" & then in the eve came a telephone message from the W.O. [War Office] that he had died at noon. We shall take up our shattered life & do the best we can. All our other dear children among whom are you dears, will be a consolation. A little letter came from my darling [Muriel]— to whom give a love & twenty kisses & some to the dear boy [Palmer].
                    Your loving Docie O."
Osler and his remarkably strong and supportive wife kept at

their appointed tasks. The perceptive among their close associates recognized how deeply he suffered, and confessions of his broken heart may be found in letters to his intimate friends among his concerns for them. He continued his many-faceted medical professional activities. With little outward sign of sorrow, "The Open Arms" was often filled with friends serving in Britain or France, and especially the staffs of newly arrived American medical units.

Revere's possessions were returned with a note from the commander of his Battery which stirred the deep emotions of his grieving parents. Osler penned notes in books Revere had loved, and with Grace considered ways to preserve his memory. The youthful Revere's savings were small. This sum was divided between his two god-sons, as indicated by notes to each of them which were enclosed in letters to Marjorie Futcher and Campbell Howard on December 4, 1917. To Marjorie his words included: "Grace keeps up splendidly, but 'tis very hard, & the heart ache is always there. Your good man is doing splendid work. I am so glad he came over." On the same day to Campbell he began with characteristic concern about the recipient, included a brief report on the illnesses among the soldiers, and an appreciation of T. B. Futcher's contribution. Osler referred also to Colonel Birkett's reposting from France on November 8, 1917, because of an illness, the prompt cure of which allowed further service with distinction:

"It is nice to hear that you are quite well again. You must be driven to death with work. Do not over do it. All goes well here —except for the gnawing sorrow in our hearts for the dear laddie. We are distributing Revere's small savings & I will send a cheque for $500 Bk. of Montreal for Palmer. Invest it for him please.[133] Much the same type of work in the Hospitals—less Typhoid & Trench fever—but scores of nerve shock & nerve wrecks. Cliveden goes strong. Futcher is much appreciated at Orpington. Birkett comes to us next week on his way home for some months."

The enclosed notes to the five-year old Palmer Howard, and six-year old Bruce Futcher were similar:

"Dearest Bruce: Revere was your godfather and loved you very much; and we are all so sad that he has been taken away. We had hoped that he would have been a nice elder brother to you both. He has left you $500, which father will take care of and give you when you get to be Revere's age, 21. It will be nice for you to have as a memorial of your god-father—so keep it separate and when you grow up you can spend the interest every year. Your loving Docie O."[134]

Revere's interest in English literature had started as an offshoot of his love of fishing. His father had given him *The Compleat Angler* by Izaak Walton (1593–1683), who was born in the reign of Elizabeth I and lived under the Stuarts to the time of Mary and William of Orange. From this much-loved early volume, Revere's interest had grown to include a good collection of 16th and 17th century classics of English literature. To these books, Osler added his own non-medical books, by authors such as Milton and Shelley, and gave them as a memorial to the Johns Hopkins University, where they were used to establish the Tudor and Stuart Club in association with the English Department. The honorary charter members suggested by the donors included about thirty of their close relatives and friends; to name a few, Sir Edmund Osler, Mrs. H.B. Chapin, the Harvey Cushings, C.P. Howards, and T.B. Futchers. Osler's letter of February 6, 1919, to Marjorie contained information about the memorial. This had been outlined in October, 1918, to President Frank J. Goodnow, who made the following announcement on Commemoration Day, February 22, 1919:

"The Edward Revere Osler Memorial will be 'The Tudor and Stuart Club', to be composed of members of the University and of friends of the donor. It will be devoted to the promotion of good fellowship and a love of literature. It will have its own library and its own endowment, made possible by this action on the part of Dr. Sir William and Lady Osler. It is hardly necessary for me to say how deeply the University appreciates their remembrance of it. . . ."

The President's announcement followed closely the suggestions contained in the donor's letter.[135]

Osler's letter to Campbell on February 14, 1918, gave him first-hand news about his friend and slightly senior colleague Lieutenant Colonel John McCrae: " 'Twas a sad business about poor Jack McCrae—pneumonia & meningitis. He had had sharp attacks of asthma, & had not had a good winter but he had stuck at the job. . . ." He had been in charge of medicine at No. 3 Canadian General Hospital from June, 1915, until a few days before his death from pneumonia on January 28, 1918. His clinical abilities were recognized by his unexpected appointment as consultant in medicine to the British 1st Army.[136]

In this letter, Osler's family news included casual mention of Campbell's nephew, about whom he must have cabled earlier. After being wounded on two previous occasions, Arthur Howard suffered briefly on October 18, 1917, from the effects of an enemy gas attack. While Acting Captain in command of a company of the Scots Guards on November 25, 1917, shrapnel fragments penetrated his abdomen. After many weeks in a critical condition, he slowly recovered, but was then invalided from active service. Osler's remarks about their own well-being were: "We keep much the same—house full all the time and so many going and coming that we have not (fortunately) much time to think."[137]

Osler made a similar reference to their sore hearts in his April 6, 1918, letter to Marjorie Futcher. He also expressed the appreciation felt at the Canadian Headquarters in London for the fine work accomplished by her husband at the Orpington Hospital.[112]

Though wars are terrible and merciless, youthful romances still flourish. "The Open Arms" would always provide a welcome for the visitor, a shelter for the sad and weary and a glorious setting for a wedding reception. Ottilie's mother, Mrs. H. P. Wright, spent most of 1915–1918 at 64 Banbury Road, a short distance from 13 Norham Gardens. The common bonds between the parents were drawn even stronger by the deaths in battle of young William Wright and Revere. Two older Wright sons also served, and their wives and the three unmarried Wright girls were active as volunteers in war work. Phoebe Wright became engaged to Captain Reginald Fitz, a Harvard physician in France. His father was Osler's friend, R. H. Fitz, famous for his descriptions of appendicitis and pancreatitis. Their wedding reception was held on the lawn on June 19, 1918. It was a large and cheery gathering, however bruised and weary some of the older hearts may have been.[138]

Later in 1918, Grace Osler received word that both her friend Marion (Mrs. H. P.) Wright and Osler's niece, Isobel Meredith had something to tell her. She clearly guessed the secret despite the remonstrance in her letter on September 27 to Mrs. Wright in London: "Confound your secrets. They are not worth 15/6 on the Great Western Railway to me. Tell any girl you know that I— Dame Grace Osler—am the female head of the Osler family." The inevitable and very happy ending was a wedding reception on the Osler lawn on January 4, 1919, for Jean Wright and Allen Pickton Osler Meredith, a Major in the Canadian Infantry.

The sorrows of battle and the aftermath of war continued up to the longed-for Armistice on November 11, 1918, and for many months thereafter in various parts of Europe. During this time, a pandemic of influenza also struck and killed many soldiers and civilians of all ages. T. Bruce Futcher died from this when only seven years old. Osler had been on the McGill Faculty in Montreal when Marjorie's brother, Bruce Howard, died of diphtheria at the age of four. With this recollection and Revere's recent death in mind, Osler wrote on November 12, 1918 to Marjorie and Tom Futcher:

"Our hearts are just aching for you. What a calamity to have to part with that dear boy [Bruce]! We can realize your grief. Poor Grace was completely prostrated when I took your cable upstairs. . . . How I wish we were with you. Ah me! these are sad days—no peace in our hearts."

Although the Armistice was the cause of great celebration among the victors, many quietly shared Osler's lament, "no peace in our hearts".

Osler expressed his sympathy to Marjorie again on December 14, 1918, and referred also to the help Revere might have given to all the young children. In this letter he mentioned the close friends who filled "The Open Arms" during the Christmas season, and also the members of American Military Hospital units about to return home. Yet the energies and time occupied in his professional and social activities could not drown his deep sorrow. In a letter to Mabel Brewster he confessed: "There may be at last a great peace. Poor dear Isaac! Would that he could have been spared to see it. How he loathed war & all its associations! . . ."[139]

His letter to Marjorie on February 6, 1919, referring to Revere and Bruce, mentioned "the enduring sorrow", but also the hope that "the new little missus is thriving." Grace Revere Futcher was born on January 16, 1919. One may wonder what name would have been chosen by Osler's older "little missus" had this child been a boy.

CHAPTER VI

Threescore Years
and Ten

THROUGH THE WINTER and the spring of 1919 Osler was engaged in many professional and humanistic activities. Yet neither his spirits or physical powers fully recovered from the stresses and sorrows of the war. Bronchial infections troubled him from time to time during the influenza pandemic. Highlights of the period were his election to join Rudyard Kipling and John Buchan and other friends as a member of "Dr. Johnson's Club", and the meeting of the British Medical Association in London. This was arranged especially for the medical officers of the Allied Armies. Probably the most important events for him, however, were an outstanding Presidential address and the receipt of a birthday gift.

The meeting of the Classical Association was held in May, 1919, at Oxford. As its President, Osler arranged an exhibit of the most important books from his *Bibliotheca Prima* section to illustrate the development of science and medicine. He also helped to arrange an exhibit of historic scientific apparatus in storage among the Oxford Colleges. Thus, the great center of classical scholarship was prepared for his inspiration rousing address, "The Old Humanities and the New Science". Sir Frederic Kenyon, a leading classical scholar confessed: ". . . I hope it made many students of science anxious to extend their knowledge of classical literature; I know it made one student of the classics wish that he had a wider knowledge of natural science. Osler himself was a well-nigh perfect example of the union of science and the humanities, which to some of us is the ideal of educational progress; and his address embodied the whole spirit of his ideal."[(140)] Another in the audience, Dr. William Welch, remarked that no physician since the time of Thomas Linacre could have filled the presidency of the

Classical Association with such distinction. Osler sent a copy of the address to Campbell Howard who was undoubtedly pleased.

Sir William Osler's seventieth birthday on July 12, 1919 was an occasion to commemmorate by articles in the *Johns Hopkins Hospital Bulletin* and editorials in the *Lancet* and other publications. Almost one hundred and fifty of his friends and pupils wrote articles for a two volume book in his honor, *Contributions to Medical and Biological Research.* The actual publication was delayed, but to mark the occasion, Sir Clifford Allbutt presided over a group in London following a meeting of the Royal Society of Medicine. Dummy volumes with the titles and names of the contributors were presented to him with affectionate words. He read his response with deep emotion while suffering the onset of a severe respiratory infection. The contributors to the anniversary volumes included W. H. Welch, W. S. Halsted, L. F. Barker, T. B. Futcher, T. McCrae, Maude Abbott, Norman Gwyn, W. Hale-White, J. S. Haldane, C. H. Mayo, and W. J. Mayo, Charles and Dorothea Singer, and C. S. Sherrington. By a strange twist of fate, Campbell Howard's article concerned the illness which proved fatal to his beloved Chief.[141]

Osler was confined to bed with bronchopneumonia for about two weeks after the Anniversary celebration, and he wrote many letters of thanks. Then his wife and he went to St. Brelade's Bay on Jersey from August 1 to September 12. Near the end of the visit Osler began to attend to the revision of his textbook. He requested suggestions from many colleagues. Probably Campbell responded on the basis of his own thoroughly annotated copy. Osler's fatal illness, however, may have discouraged Campbell from submitting a title for the British Medical Association meeting at the end of June, 1920.

The developments in medicine at the University of Toronto and McGill need description to understand other parts of Osler's next letters to Campbell Howard on July 16 and September 8, 1919. Immediately after the war, funds from the John Eaton family allowed the Toronto Medical School to establish the first full-time clinical Department of Medicine in the British Commonwealth. Colonel Duncan Graham was appointed Professor of Medicine in charge of a modern clinic with facilities for investigation at the Toronto General Hospital. Osler was undoubtedly pleased by this progress at his first medical school. He had, however, been trying to influence the Principal, Dean Birkett, and physicians at McGill, to establish similar research clinics. J. C. Meakins, a McGill medical

graduate, had participated in valuable research on cardiorespira-
tory function with Professor J.S. Haldane. The former Professor of
Anatomy at McGill, Sir Auckland Geddes, held important posts in
the British government during the war. He had recently agreed
to return in October, 1919, as successor to Sir William Peterson as
Principal of McGill University. Peterson retired at the end of June,
1919, because of ill health. Geddes, however, did not return to
McGill. He was appointed Ambassador of Great Britain to the
United States, and Sir Arthur Currie became Principal in 1920.
Money was not available then to develop a clinic at McGill on the
lines proposed by Osler.[142]

Osler wrote to Campbell on July 16, 1919:

"We had a great birthday gathering and Allbutt made the
presentation of the volume. He is wonderful—at 83. Jared & Maggie & Donald [Howard] were there. We are having a busy time
with letters & cables &c. I took to bed after it all with a racking
bronchitis—not much fever, no signs but cough of a very irritating
character & plenty of pneumococci in the sputum. I am better
today.

"How your work has grown! I hear at intervals from Iowa men
how you have come to the top in the state. I should like to see you
back in Montreal at the old school with an up-to-date clinic at the
M.G.H. I have been trying to stir up Birkett & Martin about it.
Now with the establishment in Toronto of this new Eaton clinic
the matter becomes urgent. Some joint action between the Univ.
the R.V.H. & the M.G.H. should be taken—a new clinic established at each place. I suppose they would have to be whole time
men. Jack Meakins has been offered the chair of clin. therapeutics
at Edinboro—this I expect thro. [J.S.] Haldane with whom he has
been working—but they [McGill] will try to hold him. I wish
[Auckland] Geddes was to take hold this year. . . ."

On September 8, 1919, near the end of their stay on Jersey,
Osler wrote: "We have had a splendid rest here—such a nice spot,
rocks & sea & sands & sun & nearly six weeks of fine weather. I
do hope you will be able to come over next summer. If you do we
will take a house by the sea so that the darlings may have a good
outing. You & I can go to the B.M.A. meeting at Cambridge, which
promises to be a great affair. Let me know if you could give a paper
at the medical section. The birthday was enough to give me acute
megaloencephalitis. It was awfully good of all my friends. I hope
you got the classical association address. I am sweating over the
Text-book revision & hope to have everything ready to go to press

before the end of the year. I am rearranging the nervous system
& rewriting many sections. Let me have any special suggestions.
Jared [Howard] keeps well & was able to go every morning to the
Wandsworth General Hospital. Arthur has done well.

"I have sent a strong letter to the R V H [Royal Victoria Hospi-
tal], the M G H [Montreal General Hospital], & to the Dean of the
Faculty [Birkett] urging the arrangement of special clinics on
modern lines in Med. & Surgery. I hope something may come of
it. They need stirring up a bit. The new man in anatomy [S.E.Whit-
nall of Oxford] is A.1. I do not know the physiologist [J.Tait of
Edinburgh]. I wish they had taken [Oskar] Klotz instead of [Horst]
Oertel in Pathology—tho. O. is a very good man. Love to O.[Otti-
lie] and the darlings. We long to see them. Ever yours, W.O."

The Oslers returned to Oxford on September 12, 1919, after
W.O. had regained his weight & strength. Though the clinical
manifestations had subsided, his resistance to the ever present
viral and bacterial infections was probably impaired even more
than usual. Duties took him to Glasgow and Edinburgh. He insisted on returning home by train on the evening of September 26
and reached Newcastle the following morning when the railway
strike was in force. The 282 mile trip in a borrowed motor car was
interrupted by an uncomfortable stop at an old inn before he
reached home during the afternoon of September 28. At first there
were no unusual lower respiratory symptoms. The more serious
clinical manifestations began shortly before October 6. He had a
premonition of the fatal termination when the paroxysms of cough
were most severe later in October.[143] The worst stage seemed
over when Osler concluded another report about his condition on
November 1: "I am mending now & should be up within a week."
In a letter to A.W. Pollard on November 5, he remarked: "It has
been one of these low broncho-pneumonias so common after influenza."[144]

Osler was an experienced physician and characteristically a
difficult patient for his younger colleagues, A. G. Gibson and William Collier, with whom he was often jocular or deceptive. He
examined himself carefully, and included details in letters to many
of his medical friends, as to Campbell Howard on November 1,
1919:

"I have had a horrid attack—something like one of the old
bronchitics but much worse. *First,* four or five days of ordinary
catarrh, following a long motor ride from Newcastle where I was
held up by the strike. *2nd.* Fever 100–103° for a week, with irrita-

tive coughs—(a) incessant short coughs—(b) bouts 2 or 3 an hour of eight-12 coughs, ending in expectoration of a tenacious non-tinged sputa; and (c) paroxysms of max. intensity, like whooping cough—without the whoops. Four or five a day & leaving one very prostrate. *3rd* Fever left, cough persists—no severe bouts but an occasional one of moderate severity. *4th*. Practically no physical signs—a little impaired resonance at rt. base. *5th*. M. Catarrhalis & Pneumo. no. 3 the organisms.

"I have been in bed just a month, never before for so long, & a trained nurse! Love to O[Ottilie] & M [Miss M. Wright], if she is with you. Tell little Muriel I talk a great deal about her & old Pom pom [Palmer]. Kisses to them both. Yours affec. Wm. O."

"Dear Children, I have had a bad time I can tell you. Docci O had me making lists of people to be cabled & written to tell he was dying—but he is a little better. Yrs A.G. [Grace]"

His letter to the Futchers on November 5 was similar with such phrases as "devil of an attack—nearly blew the lid off". However, he congratulated them on their new house and the two little girls, though he still bemoaned the losses of Bruce and Revere. A few days later pleural pain appeared, and then increased fremitus and pectoriloquy at the right base. One of the last letters mailed was to Campbell on November 25, 1919:

"Not much change—about one paroxysm a day now & more expectoration—no fever. Just three over 100° & pulse good. The friction has cleared up. I told you I think of the acute pleurisy— on right side 3 weeks ago. No signs of effusion. The blooming thing started with paroxysms. I am always suspicious of the pleura with hard recurrent bouts of cough after an acute pulmonary trouble. [145] Fremitus and pect.[oriloquy] to the lower limit. Great sense of constriction & talking or movement at once brings on cough. Gen. Cond. good, p. [pulse] rarely over 65—appetite A.1. Curious attack. I am in my 9th week now. Love to you all.
Your loving Docie O."

These signs of pulmonary consolidation were replaced by those of local effusion. The dreaded complication of empyema due to hemophilus influenzae was demonstrated on December 4. Later, a pulmonary abscess developed. Until near the end he continued to scribble notes. One of the last, found at his bedside, reached from his heart to those he loved: "Nothing to worry about but leaving Grace & no Isaac to comfort her, & my inability to write letters to my dear friends & to the dear little darlings in Canada & to Marjorie's children—Muriel's—and Campbell's. W.O."[146]

The details are recorded of the aspiration of pleural fluid on December 5, and despite the best available physicians and treatments of the time, the development of empyema and pulmonary abscess with fatal termination. His wife's sister, Sue Chapin, Bill Francis and Archie Malloch were with Grace when the end came peacefully on December 29, 1919. Jeremiah A. Barondess has reviewed the clinical details recorded by the attending physician, A. G. Gibson, and the consultants' reports. Barondess concurred in the opinion that the protracted illness with empyema, from which hemophilus influenzae was isolated, constituted a characteristic course in the influenza pandemic of 1918–19.[147]

In his essay, J. G. Adami included a description of the final manifestations of Osler's illness and a list of those present at his funeral. Adami stressed that his humanity and his interest in all his colleagues and friends were the outstanding characteristics of "the greatest physician of history."[148] I will not dispute Adami's view, but refer to the large number of expressions of Osler's notable attributes in the literature.[149]

Lewellys Barker subdivided his appraisal of Osler as follows: "as student and promoter of research; as teacher; as private practitioner; Osler and public health; as organizer; as writer and as bibliophile, and Osler—the man."[150] The words of his famous colleague William Welch can not be surpassed.[151] Later Sir Geoffrey Keynes emphasized the importance of Osler as a clinician: "The Oslerian Tradition in medical advances insisted on the importance of careful and expert clinical observation coupled with wide knowledge of the symptoms of disease, these two forms of 'collecting', if you like to call them so, being coordinated to form the basis of accurate diagnosis".[152]

Sir William Osler's strong and enduring influence on the young men who spent many months, many years, as medical residents, or in a similar relationship of pupil, is abundantly evident in Cushing's biography. I would also cite the appraisal of his Chief by W. S. Thayer: "He was a great teacher. But his main strength lay in the singular and unique charm of his presence, in the sparkling brilliancy of his mind, in the rare beauty of his character and of his life, and in the example that he set to his fellows and to his students. He was a quickening spirit."[153]

A rather similar view was given by one who came under Osler's influence in Britain. Sir Arthur S. MacNalty wrote: ". . . He was specially kind to his students, helping and encouraging them as they set their steps on the arduous path of medicine. He was a

great teacher and a great clinician. He made every use of his
splendid opportunities, not to his own self-glory but for the good
of his fellow mortals and the advancement of medicine. If professorial and professional duties, and a thousand calls on his time,
prevented his making any outstanding discovery, he possessed in
the highest degree the wonderful gift of inseminating knowledge
and an aptitude for research in others. . . ."[154] Osler, the Chief,
was a powerful influence in these ways on the life of his teacher's
son, Campbell Howard.

The burial service at the Chapel of Christ Church, during a
grey afternoon on January 1, 1920, was held before a large throng
of official representatives, friends and family. His favorite copy of
Sir Thomas Browne's *Religio Medici* lay on his bier. Never more
powerful imagery was set in type than Harvey Cushing's closing
paragraph:

"And perhaps that New Year night saw, led by Revere, another
procession pass by the 'watching-chamber'—the spirits of many,
old and young—of former and modern times—of Linacre, Harvey,
and Sydenham; of John Locke, Gesner and Louis; of Bartlett,
Beaumont, and Bassett; of Johnson, Bovell, and Howard; of Mitchell, Leidy, and Stillé; of Gilman, Billings, and Trudeau; of Hutchinson, Horsley, and Payne; of the younger men his pupils who had
gone before—Jack Hewetson, MacCallum, and McCrae; and in
still greater number those youths bearing scars of wounds who
more recently had known and felt the affection and warmth of the
'Open Arms'—doubly dead in that they died so young."[155]

Many devoted friends remained across the Atlantic. Each must
have felt a crushing sense of helplessness and remorse that he or
she might have given some aid or comfort to "The Chief" or Lady
Osler, "Aunt Grace." No answer can be given. Campbell and
Ottilie Howard and their two children visited Aunt Grace during
August. At "The Open Arms" they encountered Harvey Cushing
briefly. Then, as Osler had expressed the hope in his letters, they
spent several weeks with her in a cottage by the sea. (Fig. 41)

CHAPTER VII

Campbell Howard's Later Career

CAMPBELL HOWARD'S MEDICAL EDUCATION AND CAREER were stimulated and guided by his godfather, William Osler. At the time of his "Chief's" death Campbell Howard was forty-two years of age and had been Chairman of the Department of Medicine at the University of Iowa for nine years. A solid base in the instruction of anatomy under Professor H. J. Prentiss had been expanded into the other preclinical subjects. In accordance with the initial terms of the Perkins' Law, and later amendments by the State Legislature, the University Hospital was improved and enlarged to meet the increased demand to care for crippled and sick children and adults.

At the end of World War I, and during the early post-war years, expansion took place in the existing departments of medicine, surgery, and eye, ear, nose and throat. New departments of pediatrics, psychiatry, and obstetrics and gynecology were established, while divisions of radiology, anesthesia, orthopedics, urology and others were also developed. The Children's Hospital was built to the west of the Iowa River. Other units would soon follow from the scattered old buildings where they'd been housed to the new University Medical Center complex. The construction was made possible by generous donations of funds from the Rockefeller philanthropic institutions to match the appropriations from the Iowa State Legislature. Mr. Abraham Flexner, Dr. Wallace Buttrick and others of the Rockefeller Foundation and the General Education

Board were favorably impressed with the advances in medical education and research, since the reorganization of the Iowa College of Medicine in 1910. Personal ties of trust and friendship had grown between the Rockefeller officers and Walter A. Jessup, President of the University of Iowa and W. R. Boyd, Chairman of the Finance Committee of the Iowa State Board of Education.[156]

The medical faculty included many talented and dedicated leaders during this period, such as Charles Rowan in surgery, Arthur Steindler in orthopedics and persons in other areas. Professor John McClintock, who was a member of the faculty throughout the period, paid special tribute to the leadership of Doctor Prentiss, Professor of Anatomy (1904–1931), in establishing the high standard of education, to Dean L. W. Dean (1914–1927), for his effective administration in securing legislation and the funding for the growth of the College, and to Campbell Howard (1910–1924) for developing scientific research in the College of Medicine. In John T. McClintock's words: "Dr. Howard is, I think, responsible for bringing to Iowa a spirit of scientific research which was greatly needed. He established a research division in his own department and by his own efforts made it clear that research can be carried on without sacrifice to a high standard of teaching. . . ."[157]

In the summer of 1924, Campbell Howard resigned his position at Iowa to return to his alma mater in Montreal, Canada. The decision was difficult for he recognized the continuing opportunities for further development of the medical department at the Iowa College, and that the clinical metabolic research with his laboratory colleague, Robert B. Gibson, Ph. D., on remissions in pernicious anemia by dietary management had reached a critical stage. These factors not withstanding, he decided to accept the offer to be Professor of Medicine at McGill University and Physician-in-Chief at the Montreal General Hospital, positions which his father had once occupied. After the inevitable interruption in his clinical and research work, Campbell Howard reestablished many of his programs at Montreal. His clinical teaching in the Oslerian manner earned the appreciation of students and residents on his medical service. The quality of his contributions to the medical literature and his participation in medical meetings brought him the presidency of the American Society for Clinical Investigation (1924)), the Association of American Physicians (1929), and the Medico-Chirurgical Society of Montreal (1935). Howard's leadership in the councils of McGill University was recognized by his re-election as a faculty representative to the University Senate during the 1930's.

Campbell Howard's ties with Iowa were maintained through the stream of Iowa medical graduates who trained in the medical and other services at the Montreal General and affiliated hospitals. He participated in the clinical program at the dedication of the new University Hospital and Medical Center at Iowa City in November, 1928, and he was the guest speaker at the Iowa State Medical Society Meeting in Des Moines in May, 1931. His friendship with his former surgical colleague, Professor Charles J. Rowan, led him to accept the invitation to participate in meetings and give lectures at the University of Southern California at Los Angeles. Despite symptoms of phlebitis in his calf, he traveled to California and completed his duties. Painful swelling of his leg confined him to bed in his friend's home where a massive pulmonary embolism from femoral thrombophlebitis resulted in his sudden death, at the age of fifty-nine, on June 3, 1936.

Conspicuous among the mourners at the funeral in Montreal were his successive medical residents at the Montreal General Hospital, McGill students and faculty colleagues, Doctors Rowan from California and H.L. Beye, a close friend and official representative from the University of Iowa. Temporary illness prevented another from attending the funeral, but William R. Boyd whose bonds with Campbell Howard had remained strong since 1910, summarized his personal feelings about his departed friend: "His coming to Iowa City marked an epoch; he brought into the faculty a spirit of nobility sadly needed. He stood without compromise for standards that were as high as the highest. More than anyone else, he helped to 'renew a right spirit within' the College of Medicine. Later, he was joined by Dr. Rowan and others. He was as tall mentally and spiritually as he was physically, and the influence he exerted, let us hope, will be 'lines of influence which will stretch out forever'. I think they will. . . ."[158] Tributes by Dr. Howard Beye of the University of Iowa and Dr. A. H. Gordon and Dean Charles F. Martin of McGill were published in the *Canadian Medical Association Journal,* and memorial tablets were placed in the University of Iowa Hospital, and the Montreal General Hospital by his former medical colleagues and residents.[159]

Footnotes

1.   Harvey Cushing, *The Life of Sir William Osler*, 2 vols. (Oxford: Clarendon Press, 1925), I, p. 70, cited hereafter as Cushing, *Life*, I or II.

2.   Edward H. Bensley, "Robert Palmer Howard", *Dictionary of Canadian Biography/Dictionnaire Biographique du Canada* (University of Toronto Press), XI (1982), pp. 428–29.

3.   This letter is ascribed to August 2 or 3, 1876, because Osler was best man at the wedding of Dr. James Kerr and Laurie Jane Bell on July 26, 1876 (R. Mitchell and T.K. Thorlakson, *Canadian Journal of Surgery*, 9 (1966), pp. 213–14). Presumably he had sent Howard a copy of the current *Ontario Medical Register . . . with Act* (1874), but the "enclosed report" may have concerned other mutual interests. Osler's "Haemorrhagic small-pox" appeared in *Canada Medical and Surgical Journal*, 5(1877), pp. 289–304.

4.   W. Osler, "Report from Canada", *Annual Reports on the Diseases of the Chest* under the direction of Horace Dobell, 1875–76 (London: II, 1876), pp. 1–12. Osler also submitted the Canadian review for the third and last year of the series. Howard, who had contributed the article for 1874–75, remained on the editor's Board of Coadjutors for all three volumes.

5.   E.J.A. Rogers, quoted in Cushing, *Life*, I, p. 172.

6.   R.P. Howard, "Cases of Leucocythemia", *Montreal General Hospital Reports, Clinical and Pathological* (Montreal, 1880), pp. 1–2.

7.   R.P. Howard, *Medical Faculty, McGill College, Semi-centennial Celebration . . . : A Sketch of the Life of Dr. G.W. Campbell, and A Summary of the Early History of the Faculty* (Montreal, 1882), pp. 11–13, 22–23, 44.

8.   R.P. Howard, Summer 1884, to W. Osler, Cushing, *Life*, I, pp. 223–24.

9.   W. Osler, "The Cardiac Relations of Chorea", *American Journal of Medical Sciences*, 94 (October 1887), pp. 371–86.

10.   W. Osler, "The Haematozoa of Malaria", *Transactions of Pathological Society of Philadelphia*, 13 (1887), pp. 255–76; *British Medical Journal*, i (March 12, 1887), pp. 556–62.

11.   W. Osler, "The Gulstonian Lectures on Malignant Endocarditis", *British Medical Journal*, i (March 7, 1885), pp. 467–70; (March 14, 1885), pp. 522–26; (March 21, 1885), pp. 577–79; also, *Medical News*, 46 (March 21, 1885), pp. 309–13; (March 28, 1885), pp. 337–43; (April 4, 1885), pp. 365–69.

12.   Cushing, *Life*, I, pp. 260–63, 277–78.

13.   Hobart Amory Hare, "William Osler as a Teacher and Clinician, "*Therapeutic Gazette*, 44 (March 15, 1920), pp. 160–64; also, Sir William Osler Memorial Number, Appreciations and Reminiscences, ed. by Maude E. Abbott, *Bulletin of International Association of Medical Museums . . .*, 9 (1926), pp. 212–17, cited hereafter as *Appreciations* (1926).

14.   Arnold Muirhead, *Grace Revere Osler, A Brief Memoir* (Oxford University Press, 1931), p. 18.

15.   "Smith, Donald Alexander", *Dictionary of National Biography, 1912–1921* (London: Oxford University Press, 1927), pp. 496–98; "Lord Strathcona's Gift . . ., Lord Strathcona and Mount Royal . . .," *Bulletin International Association of Medical Museums*, 5 (June 1913), pp. 11–13; Unsigned Annotation, "The Late Lord Strathcona", *Lancet* i (Jan. 24, 1914), p. 255; Cushing, *Life*, I, pp. 187n, 210; *ibid.*, II, pp. 45–47, 60, 67, 70, 186, 208, 291, 303, 369, 372, 396; "R.J.B. Howard, B.A., M.D., F.R.C.S.", *Canadian Medical Association Journal*, 2 (April 1921), pp. 279–80.

16.   W. Osler, "The Student Life" in *Aequanimitas* with Other Addresses, 3rd ed. (Philadelphia: P. Blakiston's Son & Co., 1932), pp. 420–21; [Editorial] ". . . death of Dr. Palmer Howard . . . ," *Medical News* (Philadelphia), 54 (April 6, 1889), p. 383; "Robert Palmer Howard, M.D.", *ibid.* (April 13, 1889), p. 419.

17.   Sir William Dawson, April 2, 1889, to Mrs. R.P. Howard, from a scrap book which also contains "Death of Dr. Howard", *Montreal Herald and Commercial Gazette*, March 29, 1889, and other contemporary papers.

18.   This letter was published with minor editorial changes in Cushing, *Life*, I, p. 459. Letters included in *The Life* are indicated in the footnotes to the "Dates of Communications from Grace and William Osler in Appendix E.

19.   W. Osler, The Master-word in Medicine, (Baltimore, 1903); also in *British Medical Journal*, ii (November 7, 1903), pp. 1196–1200; and in the first and later editions of *Aequanimitas with Other Addresses*.

20.   Alan M. Chesney, *The Johns Hopkins Hospital and the Johns Hopkins University School of Medicine, A Chronicle*, 3 vols. (Baltimore: Johns Hopkins Press, 1943, 1958, 1963) (hereafter cited as *Johns Hopkins*, I, II or III), Thomas B. Turner, *Heritage of Excellence: The Johns Hopkins Medical Institutions, 1914–1947* (Baltimore: Johns Hopkins University Press, 1974).

21.   Simon Flexner and James T. Flexner, *William Henry Welch and the Heroic Age of American Medicine* (New York: Viking Press, 1941).

22.   William G. MacCallum, *William Stewart Halsted, Surgeon* (Baltimore: Johns Hopkins Press, 1930); G. Rainey Williams, "An Introduction to William Stewart Halsted", *Journal of the Oklahoma State Medical Association*, 64 (December 1971), pp. 488–92.

23.   W. Osler, *The Principles and Practice of Medicine* (New York: D. Appleton and Company, 1892).

24.   George T. Harrell, "Lady Osler", *Bulletin of the History of Medicine*, 53 (Spring 1979), pp. 81–99.

25.   Edith Gittings Reid, *The Great Physician, A Short Life of Sir William Osler* (New York: Oxford University Press, 1931).

26.   Thomas E. Keys, "Edward Revere Osler, 1895–1917", *Archives of Internal Medicine*, 114 (August 1964), pp. 284–93; George T. Harrell, "The Oslers' Son—Revere", *Bulletin of the History of Medicine*, 54 (Winter 1980), pp. 561–71.

27.   Reid, *The Great Physician*, p. 105.

28.   Joseph H. Pratt, "Osler as his students knew him", *Boston Medical & Surgical Journal*, 182 (April 1, 1920), pp. 338–41; *A Year with Osler, 1896–97* (Baltimore: The Johns Hopkins Press, 1949).

29.   Earl F. Nation and John P. McGovern, *Student and Chief: The Osler-Camac Correspondence . . .*, Medical Library of the Los Angeles County Medical Association, 1980.

30.   Cushing, *Life*, I, pp. 124, 127; II, 412.

31.   Chesney, *Johns Hopkins*, II

32.   Cushing, *Life*, I, p. 637.

33.   *Ibid.*, p. 645.

34.   *Ibid.*, p. 166.

35.   *Ibid.*, pp. 647–48; Scrapbook of T. Archibald Malloch, Osler Library [hereafter, O.L.], Accession No. 326/40/45; H. Cushing, "William Osler, The Man", *Annals of Medical History*, 2 (June, 1919), pp. 163–64.

36.   Cushing, *Life*, I, pp. 649–50.

37.   *Ibid.*, p. 651.

38.   W. Osler, *Aequanimitas with Other Addresses*, ed. 2, 1906, Preface and Chapter XIX.

39.   *Ibid.*, Chapter XX; Cushing, *Life*, I, pp. 675–77.

40.   Osler, *Aequanimitas . . .*, ed. 2, Chapter XXII, L'Envoi, final page.

41.   Campbell P. Howard, "The Incidence of Gastric Ulcer in America", *Medical News*, 85 (October 8, 1904), pp. 673–75; "A Study of Ulcer of the Stomach and Duodenum: Based Upon a Series of Eighty-Two Cases, "*American Journal of the Medical Sciences*, 128 (December, 1904), pp. 939–66; "Gastric Ulcer: Clinical Varieties and Symptoms", *Johns Hopkins Hospital Bulletin*, 16 (March, 1905), p. 116; "Symptomatology and Diagnosis of Gastric Ulcer", *Proceedings of the Philadelphia County Medical Society*, 26 (1905), pp. 125–31; "Gastric Tetany", *Johns Hopkins Hospital Bulletin*, 16 (April, 1905), p. 148.

42.   Cushing, *Life*, I, p. 674.

43.   "Osler in Washington", *The Sun* [Baltimore], May 17, 1905, p. 2, col. 5; Cushing, *Life*, I, pp. 681–85; *ibid.*, II, pp. 3–4.

44.   William Collier, "Sir William Osler's Work at the Radcliffe Infirmary and for the Prevention of Tuberculosis", *Appreciations* (1926), pp. 356–59. A.H.T. Robb-Smith, *A Short History of the Radcliffe Infirmary* (Oxford: United Oxford Hospitals, 1970), pp. 113–37, 209.

45. Robb-Smith, *ibid.*, pp. 113–37, 140, 143–44, 209; A. G. Gibson, "Sir William Osler at Oxford", *Appreciations* (1926), pp. 378–80; Charles Singer, "William Osler", *British Medical Journal*, i (January 3, 1920), pp. 31–32; Archibald Malloch, "Sir William Osler at Oxford", *Appreciations* (1926), pp. 363–67; E. H. Bensley, "Thomas Archibald Malloch (1887–1953)", *Osler Library Newsletter*, McGill University, Montreal, No. 36 (February 1981); Bensley, "Sir William Osler and Mabel Purefoy Fitzgerald", *ibid.*, No. 27 (February 1978); Edward S. Martin, *Abroad with Jane* (Boston: The Merrymount Press, 1918), p. 111.

46. Clifford Allbutt, "Proem: William Osler", *Appreciations* (1926), pp. xiii-xviii.

47. Cushing, *Life*, II, p. 478.

48. W. Osler, *Evolution of Modern Medicine* (New Haven: Yale University Press, 1921).

49. Cushing, *Life*, II, p. 50; W. Osler, "A Clinical Lecture on Abdominal Tumors Associated with Disease of the Testicle", *Lancet*, i (May 25, 1907), pp. 1409–12. No article by Osler on this subject has been located in Keen's *System*.

50. W. Osler, "Aneurysm of the Abdominal Aorta," *Lancet*, ii (October 14, 1905), pp. 1089–96.

51. Cushing, *Life*, II, pp. 9, 18, 128–29; "The Sargent Portrait", *ibid.*, facing p. 50.

52. *Ibid.*, pp. 18, 26; copy of Grace R. Osler's will, February 7, 1925, O.L., accession number 326/1.5.

53. C. P. Howard, "Tetany: A Report of Nine Cases", *American Journal of Medical Sciences*, 131 (February 1906), pp. 301–29.

54. C. P. Howard, "Mikulicz's Disease and Allied Conditions," *International Clinics*, 1 (1909), pp. 13–64.

55. Cushing, *Life*, II, pp. 40–41.

56. *Ibid.*, pp. 47–48; *Verhandlungen des Kongresses für innere Medezin*, 22 (1906), pp. xxxi, xxxiii, xxxvi.

57. J. A. Chatard, "An Analytical Study of Acute Lobar Pneumonia in the Johns Hopkins Hospital, from May 15, 1889 to May 15, 1905", *Johns*

Hopkins Hospital Reports, 15 (1910), pp. 55–80; C. P. Howard, "Pneumo-coccic Arthritis", *ibid.*, pp. 229–45.

58.   C. P. Howard, "The Relation of the Eosinophilic Cells of the Blood, Peritoneum and Tissues to Various Toxins", *Journal of Medical Research*, 17 (December, 1907), pp. 237–69; *British Medical Journal*, ii (October 19, 1907), p. 1074 (abstract).

59.   Cushing, *Life*, II, pp. 55–59.

60.   W. Osler, "The Growth of Truth as Illustrated in the Discovery of the Circulation of the Blood", *Lancet*, ii (October 27, 1906), pp. 1113–20, 1151–52; *British Medical Journal*, ii (October 27, 1906), pp. 1077–84; *The Times*, October 19, 1906, p. 8 de; Cushing, *Life*, II, pp. 64–67.

61.   Cushing, *Life*, II, pp. 72–77.

62.   *Ibid.*, 103; A. Malloch, "Sir William Osler at Oxford", *Appreciations* (1926), p. 374.

63.   W. Peterson, February 4, 1907, to W. Osler, enclosing report of a professorial committee of the Medical Faculty, McGill University Archives; Office of Principal W. Peterson, Correspondence; W. Osler, February 15, 1907, to Peterson, *ibid.*

64.   Dean T. G. Roddick and Principal W. Peterson, April 16–30, 1907, to Lord Strathcona, McGill University Archives; Office of Principal W. Peterson, Correspondence; "Another Fire at McGill University," *The Times* (London), April 17, 1907, p. 5e; Cushing, *Life*, II, pp. 87–89.

65.   Cushing, *Life*, II, p. 186; W. Osler, July [June] 30, 1909, to F. J. Shepherd, Cushing file, O.L., and W. Osler, July 2, 1909 to C.P. Howard; *The Times* (London), July 2, 1909, p. 5c; W. Peterson, November 12, 1909, to Lord Strathcona, McGill University Archives; Office of Principal W. Peterson, Correspondence; Lord Strathcona, December 4, 1909, to Principal Peterson, and Bursar's office, December 19, 1910, to Peterson, *ibid.* W. Osler, May 11, 1911, to Peterson, *ibid.*

66.   *"Professor Muller's Visit"*, *Montreal Medical Journal*, 36 (May, 1907), pp. 330–31; Friedrich Müller, October 6, 1907, to Peterson, McGill University Archives; Office of Principal W. Peterson, Correspondence.

67.   W. Osler: "The Diagnosis of Acute Pancreatitis", *British Medical Journal*, ii (August 10, 1907), p. 323; *ibid.*, (October 26, 1907), pp. 1132–35.

68.   W. Osler, "A Clinical Lecture on Erythaemia (Polycythaemia with Cyanosis, Maladie de Vaquez)", *Lancet,* i (January 18, 1908), pp. 143–46.

69.   Cushing, *Life,* II, pp. 137–57; W. Osler, "Impressions of Paris", *Journal of the American Medical Association,* 52 (Feb. 27, 1909), pp. 701–03; *ibid.,* (Mar. 6, 1909), pp. 771–73.

70.   Cushing, *Life,* II, pp. 173–82.

71.   W. Osler, *Michael Servetus,* London, 1909; *Bulletin of Johns Hopkins Hospital,* 21 (January, 1910), pp. 1–11.

72.   W. Osler, "Old and New", *Journal of the American Medical Association,* 53 (July 3, 1909), pp. 4–8.

73.   W. Osler, "The Treatment of Disease", *British Medical Journal,* ii (July 17, 1909), pp. 185–89; editorial, *Lancet,* ii (Oct. 2, 1909), pp. 1006–07.

74.   Cushing, *Life,* II, pp. 205–06; L. M. Payne, "The Library of the Osler Club of London", *Osler Library Newsletter,* No. 29, (October, 1978).

75.   Cushing, *Life,* II, pp. 207–08; T. B. Futcher, "Dr. Osler's Renal Stones", *Archives of Internal Medicine,* 84 (July, 1949), p. 40.

76.   W. Osler, "The Lumelian Lectures on Angina Pectoris", *Lancet,* i (March 12, 1910), pp. 697–702; *ibid.,* (March 26, 1910), pp. 839–44; *ibid.,* (April 9, 1910), pp. 973–77.

77.   Cushing, *Life,* II, pp. 213, 216.

78.   W. Osler, "Dr. William H. Welch", *American Magazine,* 70 (August, 1910), pp. 456–57, 459; A. Gregg, "Dr. Welch's Influence on Medical Education", *Bulletin Johns Hopkins Hospital,* 87 (August, 1950), Supplement 2, pp. 28–36; T. B. Turner, "William H. Welch and The Heritage of Excellence", *Johns Hopkins Medical Journal,* 134 (March, 1974), pp. 168–80.

79.   Morris Fishbein, *A History of the American Medical Association, 1847–1947,* (Philadelphia; W. B. Saunders Company, 1947), pp. 891–99; Abraham Flexner, *Medical Education in the United States and Canada, A Report of the Carnegie Foundation for the Advancement of Teaching,* Bulletin No. 4, (New York City, 1910).

80.   Abraham Flexner, "State University of Iowa, Medical Department", President G. E. MacLean's correspondence, 1910, File M-2, Uni-

versity of Iowa Archives, University Libraries, Iowa City; Minutes of the
Iowa State Board of Education, December 10, 1909, p. 115, University
of Iowa Archives; Abraham Flexner, *Medical Education in the United
States and Canada . . .*, 1910, pp. 223–25; A. Flexner, *I Remember. The
Autobiography of Abraham Flexner*, (New York: Simon and Schuster,
1940), p. 127.

81.   F. J. Smith, "History of Drake University College of Medicine",
Journal of Iowa State Medical Society, 26 (May, 1936), p. 272.

82.   Carl B. Cone, "History of the State University of Iowa: The College
of Medicine", Iowa City, 1941, typescript, pp. 171–72; *ibid.*, Appendix B,
W. R. Boyd, "A Brief History of the Development of the College of
Medicine of the Iowa State University [Iowa City]; From 1908 to Date
(1934)", pp. 1–8, University of Iowa Archives.

83.   Minutes of Meetings of Iowa State Board of Education, May 25–26,
1910, pp. 239, 245, 257; Iowa State Board of Education, Minutes of Finance
Committee and Other Committees, July 21, 1910, p. 11; Campbell Howard,
July 19, 1910, telegram to President G. E. MacLean, President MacLean's
correspondence, 1910, File H-2; Howard, August 5, 1910, telegram to MacLean, *ibid.;* MacLean, July 28 and July 29, 1910 to Campbell Howard,
ibid., File H-3; Howard, August 3, 1910, to MacLean, *ibid.*, all of which
are in the University of Iowa Archives.

84.   William Osler, July 28, 1910, to Principal W. Peterson, McGill University Archives, Office of Principal W. Peterson, Correspondence; Peterson, September 24, 1910, to William Osler, *ibid.*

85.   Cushing, *Life*, II, pp. 239, 250; Mrs. Leo S. Apedaile provided
information about the camp, with the help of Donald Ross of Quebec.

86.   James H. Breasted, *A History of Egypt; From the Earliest Times
to the Persian Conquest* (New York, Charles Scribner's Sons, 1909), pp.
156–60, 280, Fig. 168; other details of Osler's experiencesinEgyptarein
Cushing,*Life*, II, pp. 262–68.

87.   William Osler, March 1, 5 and 22, 1911, to W.S. Thayer, H. M.
Thomas, and T. McCrae, Cushing file, O.L.; Cushing, *Life*, II, pp. 263, 266,
268.

88.   One photograph shows the Osler party dining on the *Seti* (figure
28). The other photograph shows a small Nile cargoboat with two triangu-
lar sails, as Osler described in his letter to S. Weir Mitchell in Cushing,
Life, II, pp. 264–65.

89.   Cushing, *Life,* II, pp. 277–78, 291–93.

90.   W. Osler, "Whole-time Clinical Professors at the Johns Hopkins Medical School," *British Medical Journal,* ii (November 8, 1913), pp. 1242–43; W.H.W., *ibid.,* (November 15, 1913), p. 1330; Cushing, *Life,* II, pp. 382–83.

91.   Cushing, *Life,* II, pp. 272–73, 275–78.

92.   *British Medical Journal,* ii (August 5, 1911), pp. 266, 277; *ibid.,* (October 7, 1911), pp. 799–800, 820; *Lancet,* ii (August 5, 1911), p. 371; Cushing, *Life,* II, p. 286.

93.   William Osler, August 15, 1911, to W. G. MacCallum, cited in Cushing, *Life,* II, p. 290.

94.   Revere's engineering success is also recorded in Cushing, *Life,* II, p. 306.

95.   H. B. Jacobs in reply to H. Cushing's inquiry, August 27, 1923, in Cushing file, O.L., April, 1912; Cushing, *Life,* II, pp. 309–13.

96.   Grace R. Osler, January 8, [1912], to Peterson, McGill University Archives, but, Office of Principal Peterson, Correspondence.

97.   Louis Baumann and C. P. Howard, "Metabolism of Scurvy in an Adult," *Archives of Internal Medicine,* 9 (June 1912), pp. 665–79; also *Transactions of the Association of American Physicians,* 27 (1912), pp. 514–23.

98.   Cushing, *Life,* II, pp. 327–32.

99.   The Atlantic City Session, *Journal of the American Medical Association,* 58 (May 4, 1912), pp. 1363, 1371; Thomas B. Futcher, "Recent Advances in Our Knowledge Concerning the Causes of Glycosuria", *ibid.,* 59 (December 21, 1912), pp. 2238–41.

100.   W. Osler, "Specialism in the General Hospital", *Bulletin of the Johns Hopkins Hospital* 24 (June, 1913), pp. 167–71; "Dr. Osler Pays Calls", *The Sun* (Baltimore), April 16, 1913, p. 14, col. 3, et seq.; Cushing, *Life,* II, pp. 128, 349–53.

101.   "Live To-day, Says Osler", *New York Times,* April 21, 1913, p. 2, col. 2; W. Osler, *A Way of Life,* (London: Constable & Co., 1913), and elsewhere.

102.   W. Osler, "Burton's Anatomy of Melancholy", *Yale Review*, 3 (Fall, 1913), pp. 251–71; W. Osler, *Evolution of Modern Medicine*, (New Haven: Yale University Press, 1921); Cushing, *Life*, II, pp. 353–59.

103.   Cushing, *Life*, II, p. 361; W. Osler, Commencement Address, *Johns Hopkins Hospital Nurses' Alumnae Magazine*, 12 (July, 1913), pp. 72–81; Dr. Osler to Nurses, *The Sun* (Baltimore), May 8, 1913, p. 4, col. 3–4.

104.   Muirhead, *Grace Revere Osler*, previously cited, pp. 26, 54; Margaret Revere, personal letter.

105.   Cushing, *Life*, II, pp. 365, 400, 446; Cushing, Chronological File, 1913, O.L.

106.   Annotation, "The Late Lord Strathcona", *Lancet*, i (January 24, 1914), p. 255; "Lord Strathcona and Mount Royal . . .", *Bulletin of the International Association of Medical Museums*, 5 (June 1915), pp. 12–13; Cushing, *Life*, II, pp. 372, 396.

107.   Cushing, *Life*, II, pp. 312, 392, 397.

108.   E. H. Bensley and D. G. Bates, "Osler's Autobiographical Notes", *Bulletin of the History of Medicine*, 50 (Winter, 1976), p. 617; M. Fransiszyn, Osler Library, McGill, January 29, 1979, personal communication.

109.   Cushing, *Life*, II, pp. 292–93, 382–83; W.O., May 23, 1911, to Campbell Howard; Chesney, *Johns Hopkins*, III, pp. 244–62; T. B. Turner, *Heritage of Excellence, The Johns Hopkins Medical Institutions*, 1914–1947 (Baltimore: The Johns Hopkins University Press, 1974), pp. 105–08.

110.   C. P. Howard, "The Etiology and Pathogenesis of Bronchiectasis", *American Journal of Medical Sciences*, 147 (March, 1914), pp. 313–32; *Transactions of the Association of American Physicians*, 28 (1913), pp. 758–80. No publication by William Osler has been identified which included his own recent observations.

111.   Francis A. Winter, "Sir William Osler and the American Medical Officer", *Contributions to Medical and Biological Research Dedicated to Sir William Osler . . .* , (New York: Paul B. Hoeber, 1919), Vol. II, pp. 1267–68; Cushing, *Life*, II, pp. 525, 528, 569–70.

112.   W.A.B. Douglas, Director of History, National Defense Headquarters, Ottawa, April 2, 1979, file 1325–500/H; "Army Medical Services," *Canadian Medical Association Journal*, 7 (October, 1917), p. 950; Cushing, *Life*, II, p. 588.

113. W. Osler, "Looking Back", *Bulletin Johns Hopkins Hospital,* 25 (December 1914), pp. 354–55.

114. Cushing, *Life,* II, pp. 431–37.

115. A. H.T. Robb-Smith, *A Short History of the Radcliffe Infirmary,* (Oxford, 1970), pp. 132–34.

116. Cushing, *Life,* II, pp. 467, 477–80.

117. *Ibid.,* pp. 479–81, 483, 486–87; John McCrae, *In Flanders Fields and Other Poems,* (London and New York: G. P. Putnam's Sons, 1919).

118. C. P. Howard, "The Diagnosis of Mediastinitis", *Johns Hopkins Hospital Bulletin,* 26 (May, 1915), pp. 140–44; "Annotation", *Lancet,* ii (August 14, 1915), pp. 350–51; Cushing, *Life,* II, pp. 426, 430, 497, 517–18; W. L. Brown, "Discussion on Trench Nephritis", *Proceedings, Royal Society of Medicine,* 9, pt. 2 (February 15, 1916), pp. i-xl, including Osler's discussion on pp. xiv-xvii.

119. "Dr. Charles J. Rowan . . . ," *Daily Iowan,* January 6, 1914, p.1, col.3; Berkeley Moynihan, "John B. Murphy—Surgeon", *Surgery, Gynecology and Obstetrics,* 31 (December, 1920), pp. 549–73; Deaths: John Benjamin Murphy, M.D., *Journal of the American Medical Association,* 67 (August 19, 1916), p. 629.

120. Cushing, *Life,* II, pp. 486–87, 495, 499–500; C.P. Howard, "Recollections of Sir William Osler's Visit . . . ," *Appreciations* (1926), pp. 419–20.

121. W.O., November 15[?], 1915, to Principal Peterson, McGill University Archives, Office of Principal W. Peterson, Correspondence; "Van Epps Takes Howard's Place", *Daily Iowan,* February 24, 1915, p. 1, col.5; Minutes of the Meetings of the Iowa State Board of Education, Finance Committee and Other Committees, March 31, 1915, pp. 323–31; *ibid.,* August 31, 1915, pp. 119–21, Iowa U. Archives; *Report of the Iowa State Board of Education for the Biennial Period Ending June 30, 1916,* pp. 7–21, 55, 121, 139; "Hospital Facilities are Taxed", *Daily Iowan,* February 5, 1916, p. 1, col. 2

122. W. Peterson, Dec. 6, 1915, to W. Osler, McGill University Archives, Office of Principal W. Peterson Correspondence; Peterson, Nov. 30, 1915, to the Honorable Sir Sam Hughes. Peterson, Dec. 1, 1915, to Major Howard, Howard, Nov. 15, 1915, to Peterson; Hughes, December 2, 1915, to Peterson, *ibid.*

123.   "Howard Describes Service at Front . . .," *Daily Iowan,* February
9, 1916, p. 1, col. 1–2; "Dr. Howard", *ibid.,* February 9, 1916, p. 4, col. 2;
"Dr. Howard Speaks at Joint Meeting", *ibid.,* December 15, 1917, p. 1,
col.3.

124.   Minutes of the Meetings of the Faculty of Medicine, June 7, 1915,
and January 29, 1916; Minutes of the Meetings of the Iowa State Board of
Education Finance Committee on November 18, 1915, and February 25,
1916, pp. 213, 311; Minutes of the Board of Education on March 8, 1916, pp.
315–17, all of which are in the University of Iowa Archives.

125.   Cushing, *Life,* II, pp. 510, 530.

126.   *Ibid.,* pp. 519–20.

127.   *Ibid.,* pp. 542–43.

128.   *Ibid.,* pp. 536–39; "Canadian Army Medical Service; Report of
the Board of Inquiry", *British Medical Journal,* i (January 6, 1917), pp.
16–20.

129.   R. P. Strong, *Trench Fever, Report . . ., American Red Cross,*
(Oxford University Press, 1918); review by W. Osler, *Lancet,* ii (October
12, 1918), pp. 496–98; Cushing, *Life,* II, pp. 610–12, 621–22.

130.   Cushing, *Life,* II, pp. 523, 529, 613; J. C. Meakins, J. Parkinson, E.
B. Gunson, T. F. Cotton, J. G. Slade, A. N. Drury, and T. Lewis, "Heart
Affections in Soldiers, with special reference to prognosis of 'irritable
heart' ", *British Medical Journal,* ii (Sept. 23, 1916), pp. 418–20.

131.   Cushing, *Life,* II, pp. 546–50, 568–69.

132.   *Ibid.,* pp. 576–78; H. Cushing, *From a Surgeon's Journal, 1915–
1918,* (Boston: Little, Brown and Company, 1936), pp. 197–98, 296; John F.
Fulton, *Harvey Cushing; A Biography,* (Springfield, Illinois: Charles C.
Thomas, 1946), pp. 425–26.

133.   A major part of this letter was incorrectly cited under April 11,
1918 in Cushing, *Life,* II, p. 598.

134.   For the letter to Palmer Howard, see *ibid.,* p. 587.

135.   "Commemoration Day, 1919", *Johns Hopkins University Circu-
lar,* 38 (1919), pp. 71–72; "Annual Report of the President", *ibid.,* p. 1207;
"Letter addressed by the founders to the President of the University",

The Book of the Tudor and Stuart Club of the Johns Hopkins University, (1927), pp. 5–6; Cushing, *Life*, II, p. 630.

136.   Note 116; "Editorial, Lieutenant Colonel John McCrae . . . ," *Canadian Medical Association Journal*, 8 (March, 1918), pp. 243–47; "Obiturary, John McCrae, M.D.," *British Medical Journal*, i (February 9, 1918), pp. 190–92; Cushing, *Life*, II, p. 593.

137.   Cushing, *Life*, II, pp. 593–95.

138.   *Ibid.*, pp. 598, 607.

139.   *Ibid.*, pp. 625–27.

140.   *Ibid.*, pp. 648–49; W. Osler, "The Old Humanities and the New Science", *British Medical Journal*, ii (July 5, 1919), pp. 1–7.

141.   C. P. Howard, "The Clinical Aspects of the Pneumonia of Influenza", *Contributions to Medical and Biological Research Dedicated to Sir William Osler, Bart., M.D., F.R.S. in Honour of His Seventieth Birthday, July 12, 1919*, 2 vols., (New York: Paul B. Hoeber, 1919), Vol. I, pp. 575–81; Cushing, *Life*, II, pp. 659–61.

142.   William Osler, April 25, 1919, to F. J. Shepherd, cited in Cushing, *Life*, II, 647; *ibid.*, pp. 664–65; "Sir Auckland Geddes", *British Medical Journal*, i (April 12, 1919), 463; "Physician as British Ambassador", *Journal of the American Medical Association*, 74 (March 6, 1920), p. 684.

143.   Cushing, *Life*, II, pp. 669–71.

144.   *Ibid.*, p. 672.

145.   This sentence and "curious attack" were cited, *ibid.*, p. 679.

146.   *Ibid.*, p. 683.

147.   *Ibid.*, pp. 680–85; J.A. Barondess, "A Case of Empyema: Notes on the Last Illness of Sir William Osler," *Transactions of the American Clinical and Climatological Association*, 86 (1975), pp. 59–72.

148.   J. George Adami, "Sir William Osler: The Last Days", *Appreciations* (1926), pp. 421–28.

149.   E. F. Nation, C. G. Roland, and J. P. McGovern, *An Annotated Checklist of Osleriana*, (Kent, Ohio: Kent State University Press, 1976).

150.   L. F. Barker, "Osler in America: With Especial Reference to His Baltimore Period", *Canadian Medical Association Journal*, 33 (October, 1935), pp. 353–59.

151.   William H. Welch, "Foreword", *Appreciations* (1926), pp. i-xi.

152.   Geoffrey Keynes, "The Osler Tradition", *British Medical Journal*, 4 (December 7, 1968); p. 601.

153.   W. S. Thayer, "Osler", *Appreciations* (1926), p. 293.

154.   A. S. MacNalty, "Some Reminiscences of Osler", *Medical Press*, No. 5749 (July 13, 1949); p. 29.

155.   Cushing, *Life* II, p. 686; Edgar A. Poe mourned for his wife, "doubly dead in that she died so young, in his poem, "Lenore," 1843.

156.   A. Flexner, *I Remember . . .* , pp. 291–95; *The Rockefeller Foundation: Annual Report, 1922* (New York: The Rockefeller Foundation), pp. 346–49.

157.   C. B. Cone, "History of the State University of Iowa . . .", Appendix C., John T. McClintock, September 26, 1944, to Dean C. E. Seashore, Graduate College, pp. 1–2, Iowa U. Archives.

158.   W. R. Boyd, June 6, 1936, to Mrs. C. P. Howard, Muriel and Palmer Howard, personal collection.

159.   W. L. Bierring, *A History of the Department of Internal Medicine: State University of Iowa College of Medicine, 1870–1958*, (Iowa City: Iowa U. Press, 1958) pp. 52–61; H.E. MacDermot, *A History of the Montreal General Hospital* (Montreal, 1950), pp. 115–16, 118; C. F. Martin, "Dr. Campbell Palmer Howard", *Canadian Medical Association Journal*, 35 (July, 1936), pp. 78–79; Obituaries, "Dr. Campbell P. Howard" with appreciations by A. H. Gordon, McGill University, and H. L. Beye, State University of Iowa, *ibid.*, p. 104.

Biographical Notes

Abbott, Maude E. (1869–1920). M D, Bishop's University, Montreal, 1905; LL D, McGill. Assistant Professor of Pathology, McGill. She classified Osler's pathological specimens which remained at the McGill Medical Museum. This initiated her classical work, *Atlas of Congenital Cardiac Disease* (New York, 1936). She composed a bibliography of Osler's writings and edited the Memorial Volume, *Bulletin of the International Association of Medical Museums* 9, 1926.

Adami, J. George (1862–1926). LL D; Fellow of Royal Society. Earned natural science and medical degrees and trained in comparative pathology at Cambridge. Also trained in Europe. Professor of Pathology, McGill University, 1892–1918, including World War I service in the Canadian Army Medical Corps. He attained rank of Colonel with administrative duties. He was Vice-Chancellor, University of Liverpool, 1919–26. Adami was President of the Association of American Physicians, 1912, and lectured on the Study of Evolution in 1917 at the Royal College of Physicians. His *Principles of Pathology* (1909), and textbook with J. McCrae at McGill (1913), provided a clear exposition of this bioscience.

Allbutt, Sir Thomas Clifford (1836–1925). M B, 1861, M D, Cambridge, 1869. FRS, LL D; knighted in 1907. He trained at St. George's Hospital, London, and practiced in Leeds until

1889. He was Regius Professor of Physic [Medicine], Cambridge, from 1892–1925, and president of British Medical Association, 1916–21. Wrote *System of Medicine* (8 vols., 1896–1899; 2nd edition, 1905–12); and *Disease of the Arteries and Angina Pectoris* (1918). His Harveian Oration "Science and Medieval Thought" and other published lectures revealed his classical and historical scholarship.

Aschoff, Ludwig (1866–1942). M D, Strasburg. Professor of Pathology at Marburg, 1903–06 and Freiburg, 1906–36. Author of many books, including one on pathological anatomy and histology with H.R. Gaylord in German and English editions (1900–01), and *Lehrbuch der pathologischen Anatomie* (Jena, 1909).

Asquith, Herbert Henry (1852–1928). British Liberal politician and Prime Minister, 1908–1916.

Babinski, Joseph (1857–1932). Paris physician, pupil of Charcot. He became Chief of the Medical Service at Hôspital La Pitié. He described several reflexes useful in clinical diagnosis, and gained international fame as a neurologist.

Baker, Susan Revere (c. 1901–c. 1960). Daughter of Mr. and Mrs. R. Baker of Canton and Boston. They named her after their friend, Mrs. John Revere. The Oslers met the Bakers in December, 1908, in Paris and again in Rome during February, 1909. Osler was devoted to this young girl, and her doll, "Rosalie", the object of many make-believe experiences in Susan's play hours and correspondence with Osler (Cushing, *Life*, II, 161, et seq.)

Balfour, Arthur J., Earl of Balfour (1848–1930). British Conservative Party politician. Prime Minister, 1902–05.

Barker, Lewellys F. (1867–1943). M B, Toronto, 1890; LL D, Toronto, 1905 and others. He studied one year under William Osler. As Assistant Resident Pathologist, 1892–99, Johns Hopkins Hospital, he worked under W. H. Welch and F. P. Mall. Professor of Anatomy, University of Chicago, 1900–05, including a year of clinical research in Germany. He succeeded Osler in 1905 as Professor of Medicine at Johns Hopkins, where he established clinical research laboratories, while stressing that the individual patient be considered a psychobiological unit. He declined to become full-time professor at Johns Hopkins in 1914, but continued private practice and Clinical Professorship. Wrote important medical books and articles.

Barondess, Jeremiah A. (1924–   ). M D, Johns Hopkins, 1949. Attending physician, New York Hospital; President, American College of Physicians, 1978–79.

Bartlett, Elisha (1804–1855). M D, Brown, 1826. After training by Rhode Island practitioners and medical lecturers, he received his degree. The next year he studied under the famous Parisian clinicians, Laënnec and Louis, before starting medical practice in Lowell, Massachusetts. Soon he began a career of teaching during the winter sessions at various medical schools in the East, Kentucky, and lastly, New York City. An able clinician, teacher, and editor, his fame rests mainly on his writings, especially his book on *Fevers* (1842 and later editions), in which typhoid fever is clearly delineated from typhus. Osler published a biographical address, "Elisha Bartlett, A Rhode Island Philosopher" (1899).

Bassett, John Y. (1805–1851). M D, Washington Medical College. Practitioner in Huntsville, Alabama, who left his practice and family in December, 1835, to study in Edinburgh and Paris, where he remained through October, 1836. Later, he published articles on the diseases in his Alabama region. Osler commented on his life and writings in "An Alabama Student" (1896), and also in his book of essays with the same title (1908).

Baumann, Louis (1880–1954). M D, Columbia, New York, 1901. Assistant Professor and in charge of the research laboratory, Department of Theory and Practice of Medicine, State University of Iowa, 1911–1918. He published biochemical findings in animal and human studies, often with C.P. Howard. From 1919–1946, he contributed in biochemistry to the Departments of Medicine and Surgery, Presbyterian Hospital-Columbia University, New York City.

Beaumont, William (1785–1853). Licensed 1812; M D (Hon), 1833. While U.S. Army surgeon stationed at Fort Mackinac near Sault Ste. Marie in 1822, he treated a Canadian voyageur (St. Martin) for a gastric fistula from an accidental gunshot wound. Thus, he pursued original studies of digestion and stomach movement. Not only did he identify hydrochloric acid in the gastric juice, but he noted changes in the appearance of the stomach during ingestion, mechanical stimulation or emotional stresses. Later Beaumont was a successful practitioner in St. Louis. Beaumont's book, *Experiments and Observations of the Gastric Juice and the Physiology of Digestion* (1833), is regarded as an outstanding American contribution to medical science in the 19th century. Osler's address, "William Beaumont. A Pioneer American Physiologist" (1902), was reprinted in *An Alabama Student* (1908), and also as a preface to a reprint of Beaumont's book.

Behring, Emil von (1854–1917). German physician, a pupil of R. Koch. With Kitsato in Koch's Institute, Berlin, he developed antitoxin by immunizing animals with attenuated diphtheria toxin, 1890–1893. During 1894, antitoxin became available for general use in man.

Bethune, Elsie, of Toronto. A friend of Amo (Mrs. Wilmot) Matthews.

Bevan, Arthur D. (1861–1943). M D, Rush, 1883. After training he was associated with Rush Medical College from 1887; Professor and Head of Surgery Department, 1902–1934; also

Chief of Surgery, Presbyterian Hospital, 1894–1934. He was on the original American Medical Association Committee on Education, 1902–04; Chairman, Council on Medical Education, 1904–28, except for the years of 1917–19, when he was President-elect and President of the American Medical Association. He was a founding member and Governor of the American College of Surgeons, and President of the American Surgical Association, 1935.

Beye, Howard L. (1886–1936). M D. Rush, 1911. Trained at Cook County Hospital. His first appointment at University of Iowa was Instructor in Surgery, 1914. He was progressively promoted to Professor in 1924, and Head of the Department in 1927, which he remained until a fatal motor accident on September 29, 1936.

Bichat, Marie-Francois-Xavier (1771–1802). M.D. Famous physician of Paris who emphasized importance to pathology of tissues rather than whole organs.

Bierring, Walter L. (1868–1961). M D, Iowa, 1892. Professor of Pathology and Bacteriology, 1893–1903, and Professor of the Theory and Practice of Medicine, Iowa, 1903–1910; Professor of Internal Medicine, Drake University, Des Moines, 1910–13; Professor Emeritus of Medicine, University of Iowa, 1946–61; Iowa State Commissioner of Health, 1933–53; President of the American Medical Association, 1934–35, Alpha Omega Alpha Honor Medical Society and many others.

Billings, Frank (1854–1932). M D, Chicago Medical College, 1881; trained at Cook County Hospital and abroad; on clinical faculty, Northwestern Medical School, 1886–98; Professor of Medicine and Dean, Rush Medical College, 1899–1919. He helped organize or enlarge the University of Chicago School of Medicine, Presbyterian Hospital and many other medical institutions. He was President of the American Medical Association, 1902–04 and influential in establishment of the Council on Medical Education; President of the

Association of American Physicians, 1906. In addition to a large consulting practice, he collaborated with E. C. Rosenow on the doctrine of focal infection in sinuses, tonsils and teeth as causes of chronic illness, and edited Forchheimer's *System of Therapeutics*. He received the Distinguished Service Medal for his organizational accomplishments in World War I.

Billings, John Shaw (1838–1913). M D, Medical College of Ohio, 1860. On active duty in Civil War, 1862–64; assigned to Surgeon-General's office, 1864–95. Created U. S. Surgeon-General's Library, and initiated its Catalogue and the Index Medicus; submitted plan for Johns Hopkins Hospital in 1876, and continued as a consultant for the School of Medicine; Director of New York Public Library, 1896–1913.

Birkett, Herbert S. (1864–1942). M D, McGill, 1886; L L D, 1921. Professor of Laryngology, later, Otolaryngology, 1894–1932. Dean of Medicine, McGill, 1914–1921. Colonel, Commanding No. 3 Canadian General Hospital, 1914–1918; Brigadier General and Assistant Director General of Medical Services, Canadian Army in Europe, 1918–19.

Birks, Henry (1840–c. 1928). Founder of Henry Birks & Sons, Ltd. (Jewelers), at the turn of the 19th century. A citizen of Montreal and a leading philanthropist.

Bloodgood, Joseph C. (1867–1935). M D, Pennsylvania, 1891. Assistant Resident and Resident Surgeon, 1893–97, Johns Hopkins Hospital. Subsequently, he was Associate in Surgery at the Hospital and then Professor of Clinical Surgery, Johns Hopkins Medical School. He continued private practice in Baltimore. He was a founding member of the American Society for the Control of Cancer, Fellow of American College of Surgeons; a member of many surgical societies, the American Association for Cancer Research and the Radiological Society of North America.

Boerhaave, Hermann (1868–1738). Dutch physician who taught chemistry and botany at Leyden; then gained fame as a clinician whose bedside teaching inspired students. His pupils brought his methods to Göttingen, Vienna, Edinburgh and elsewhere.

Boggs, Thomas R. (1875–1935). M D, Johns Hopkins, 1901. House Officer and Assistant Resident under Osler and L.F. Barker to 1908, and Resident Physician, Johns Hopkins, 1908–11. Later Associate Professor of Clinical Medicine, and in private practice. Decorated for his services in U.S. Medical Corps in World War I. President of Association of American Physicians, 1937.

Borden, Sir Robert (1854–1937). Prime Minister of Canada, 1911–1920.

Bovell, James (1817–80). M.D. A native of Barbados, studied medicine in London and elsewhere in Great Britain before he practiced in Toronto, 1840–70. He taught clinical medicine at the Toronto General Hospital in various medical schools. Professor of Institutes and Dean, Trinity College Medical Faculty, 1850–56. Professor of Natural Theology, Trinity College, and Lecturer of physiology and pathology, Toronto School of Medicine, 1857–70. Bovell was medical director of Trinity College School, 1864–70 and encouraged Osler's interest in microscopy and biology while he was at the School in Weston, and College in Toronto. In 1870, Bovell returned to the West Indies and became an Anglican parish priest. He wrote *Outlines of Natural Theology for the Use of Canadian Students* (Toronto, 1859), as well as articles in Toronto medical journals.

Boyd, William R. (1864–1950). A B, University of Iowa, 1889; LL D, Iowa University and Coe College. Boyd was both Postmaster of Cedar Rapids and Editor of its newspaper, *The Republican,* for many years. In 1909, he resigned from these positions to accept chairmanship of the Finance Committee of the State Board of Education in Iowa, 1909–49. He gave "forceful leadership in Iowa higher educational affairs and [was] perhaps more responsible than any other individual for the growth and development of the medical college and hospital . . ." (*Annals of Iowa* 30: (1950), p. 391).

Brewster, Mrs. Robert (Miss Mabel Tremaine) (c. 1882–   ). Osler met her professionally in 1900 before she married Robert Brewster of New York City. After 1907, Osler corresponded frequently with her and her young daughter, Sylvia. The Oslers and Brewsters exchanged visits in New York and Oxford.

Browne, Arthur A. (1848–1910). M D, McGill, 1872. Rommate of Osler in Montreal in 1870, in London, 1872–73, and close friend thereafter. Practiced in Montreal and became Professor of Midwifery at McGill in 1882.

Browne, Sir Thomas (1605–1682). Physician of Norwich who is renowned as author of *Religio Medici* (1642), *Urn-Burial* and *Christian Morals*. Osler obtained an 1862 edition of the three principal works and other works in February, 1868. That copy was the cornerstone of his collection and he referred to it as his companion on life's road.

Buchan, John (Lord Tweedsmuir) (1875–1940). Born in Scotland, he studied at the Universities of Glasgow and Oxford. His fame rests on his historical novels and biographies. He also wrote *The History of the Great War*, and was Governor-General of Canada, 1935–40.

Burdon-Sanderson, Sir John S. (1828–1905). M D, Edinburgh, 1851. After studies in Paris, he was medical registrar at St. Mary's Hospital in 1853, and had various clinical and research positions in London. He was Professor of Physiology, University College, London, 1874–1881, and Professor of Physiology, Oxford, 1882. Appointed Regius Professor Medicine, 1894–

1904. He wrote a *Handbook for Physiological Laboratory* (1872) before Osler was his pupil in London. In 1875, he first recorded the heart beat with a capillary electrometer.

Buttrick, Wallace (1853–1926). B D, Rochester Theology Seminary, 1883; D D, Rochester University, 1898. Member, Rockefeller Foundation and related philanthropic groups; Secretary, General Education Board, 1902–17, President 1917–25.

Byers, J. Roddick (1876–1963). M D, McGill, 1902. Specialized in the treatment of tuberculosis. Served as physician at a private sanitarium in Ste. Agathe, near Montreal, before World War I, and at a similar Army installation during the War. Later reestablished his practice in Montreal.

Camac, Charles N.B. (1868–1940). M D, Pennsylvania, 1895. Assistant resident of medicine on Osler's service at Johns Hopkins, 1896–97. He then worked in the medical departments of Cornell and Columbia. He also practiced in New York until 1935, when he retired to Altadena, CA. He was a close friend of his "Chief" and Lady Osler. Wrote *Counsels and Ideals from the Writings of William Osler* (1905); 2nd edition (1921); and other historical and professional papers.

Carnegie, Andrew (1835–1919). As a boy he migrated from Scotland to Pittsburg, Pennsylvania. Without the benefit of more than a grade school education, he made his own way and earned a large fortune. In 1901, he sold his steel company to founders of U.S. Steel Corporation. He then distributed his wealth among public libraries, institutes of higher education in America and Scotland, and lay and church associations to promote world peace. Among his publications was *The Gospel of Wealth*, which shows his philosophy of philanthropy.

Carson, Major-General John W. (1864–1922). General officer commanding Canadian Forces in England, 1915–16; in command of local forces in Canada until 1918.

Cattanach, Ernest. A Canadian friend of Wilmot Matthews and
    E.B. Osler.

Chantemesse, André (1851–1919). Physician of Paris particularly
    interested in infectious disorders. With F. Widal, he intro-
    duced vaccine against typhoid fever, 1888.

Chapin, Henry B. (c.1858–1910). Massachusetts business man mar-
    ried to Susan Revere, the sister of Grace Osler.

Chapin, Susan T. (Mrs. Henry B.) (1865–1961). Sister of Grace (Re-
    vere) Osler. One son, Henry, died young. Another son, John
    R., married Margaret, whose daughter was born on May 2,
    1913.

Chatard, Joseph A. (1879–1956). M D, Johns Hopkins, 1903. Taught
    on the junior clinical staff at Johns Hopkins before and after
    World War I military service. He maintained a clinical prac-
    tice in Baltimore throughout his career.

Chauffard, Anatole (1855–1932). An able clinician who gave an
    early description of congenital hemolytic jaundice, and also
    of the syndrome associated with cancer of the tail or body
    of the pancreas.

Christian, Henry A. (1876–1951). M D, Johns Hopkins, 1900; LL D.
    Trained in Pathology and Internal Medicine at Harvard and
    its Hospitals, 1900–07. Assistant Professor of Medicine, 1907–
    08; Dean of Medicine, 1908–12; Hersey Professor of Medi-
    cine, 1908–39 and Physician-in-Chief, Peter Bent Brigham
    Hospital, 1910–39, later emeritus professor and physician.
    He was President of the Association of American Physicians
    in 1935, and received many other professional honors. He
    published one of the initial descriptions of Hand-Schuller-
    Christian syndrome (defects in membranous bones, diabe-
    tes insipidus, exophthalmos) in *Contributions to Medical*

and Biological Research, dedicated to Sir William Osler (New York, 1919) I, pp. 390–401. He revised, under his name, the 13th–16th editions of *The Principles and Practice of Medicine* (1938–1947), which Osler had originated. Christian also edited *The Oxford Medicine* and *Oxford Monographs on Diagnosis and Treatment* (both published by Oxford University Press).

Cohnheim, Julius F. (1839–1884). R. Virchow's pupil and colleague, who demonstrated that the emigration of leukocytes from the capillaries is the essential feature of inflammation. He made many outstanding contributions to pathogenesis by observations on living tissues, e.g., the development of infarction, and the infectiousness of tuberculosis through inoculation in rabbits.

Cole, Rufus (1872–1966). M D, Johns Hopkins, 1899. House Officer and Assistant Resident on Osler's medical service, 1899–1904; then Resident Physician, 1904–06, and Associate in Medicine in charge of biological laboratory in medicine at Johns Hopkins under L.S. Barker, 1906–08. From 1909 to 1937, Cole was Director of the Rockefeller Hospital and a Member of the Rockefeller Institute. He established a full-time Medical Division where clinical management and research were controlled by the resident staff under his direction. He was President of the Association of American Physicians, 1931.

Collier, William (1856–1935). M A, Cambridge, 1881; M D, 1885. House physician at Radcliffe Infirmary, 1881, and honorary attending physician, 1885–1921; thereafter, consultant and vice-president of the Infirmary. He was president of the British Medical Association when it met in Oxford in 1904. He served as Lieutenant Colonel in charge of the 3rd Southern General Hospital in Oxford during World War I.

Colwell, Nathan P. (1870–1936). M D, Rush, 1900. Secretary, Council on Medical Education and Hospitals, American Medical

Association, 1906–31. He drafted the organization documents for the Federation of State Medical Boards of the United States in 1912, and edited the bulletin, 1912–31.

Corner, Thomas Cromwell (1865–1938). Baltimore portrait painter who studied at Baltimore, New York, and Paris.

Corvisart, Jean-Nicholas (1775–1821). Leading medical clinician of Paris after the Revolution. He emphasized percussion of the chest, and wrote on diseases of the heart and lungs.

Crile, George W. (1864–1943). M D, Wooster College, 1897. Professor of Clinical Surgery, Western Reserve University, Cleveland, from 1890. Wrote on experimental studies on surgical shock, 1900; blood pressure in surgery, 1903; hemorrhage and transfusion, 1909; and the reduced mortality after operations performed under local and general anesthesia together.

Crouzon, Octave (1874–1938) Physician at Hôtel Dieu, Paris; published often on neurological disorders and also described cranial-facial dysostosis.

Currie, Sir Arthur W. (1875–1933). Served in World War I, 1914–19; General Commanding Canadian Corps in France, 1917–19. Principal, McGill University, 1920–33.

Cushing, Harvey W. (1869–1939). M D, Harvard, 1895. After interning in Boston, he was Assistant Resident one year, Resident Surgeon, 1897–1900, and Associate in Surgery, 1902–12, Johns Hopkins Hospital. He worked with the neurologist Sherrington in England, and the surgeon, Kocher, in Switzerland, 1900–02. Following his brilliant contributions to neurosurgery and endocrinology, he was appointed Professor of Surgery at Harvard and Surgeon-in-Chief, Peter Bent Brigham Hospital, 1912–32. He served with American volunteer units or with the A.E.F. in France in 1915–18, but frequently visited Allied units and Osler in Oxford. After retirement from surgical work, he was Professor of Neurology, Yale, 1933–37, and Director of Studies in History of Medicine, Yale, 1937–39. His large collection added to those of A. Klebs and J.F. Fulton formed the Historical Library, Yale Medical School. Among his publications are *The Pituitary Body and Its* Disorders (1912), *The Life of Sir William Osler* (1926), *From a Surgeon's Journal* (1937), and *Selected Papers on Neurosurgery* (1969).

Darrach, William (1876–1948). M D, Columbia, 1901. F.A.C.S. Served in U.S. Medical Corps, World War I. Surgical Director of First Division, Bellevue Hospital. Professor of Clinical Surgery through 1946, Columbia University Medical School, New York, and Dean, 1919–1930.

Dawson, Sir John William (1820–1899). Born at Pictou, Nova Scotia. Trained in Geology at Edinburgh University. Professor of Geology and Principal of McGill College, 1855–1893. Also taught biology to students in medical school. Published papers related to geology and natural history, including the theory of evolution.

Dean, Lee Wallace (1875–1944). M D, Iowa, 1896. Professor of eye, ear, nose and throat diseases, 1903–1927; Dean, College of Medicine, 1914–1927, State University of Iowa. He then served as Professor of Otolaryngology, Washington University School of Medicine, St. Louis. Fellow of the American College of Surgeons, and president of important societies in his specialty.

Delafield, Francis (1841–1913). M D, College of Physicians and Surgeons, New York, 1863. After study in Europe, he practiced and did pathology at his College; appointed Professor of Medicine, 1882. One of the founders of Association of American Physicians, 1885. He wrote *Handbook of Post-Mortem Examinations and Morbid Anatomy* (1872).

Dieulafoy, Georges (1839–1911). Physician of Paris who was a fine bedside clinician, teacher and a dramatic lecturer. He was a pioneer in the use of the trocar for the diagnosis of pleural effusions and hydatid cysts.

Drake, J. Morley (1828–1886). A Montreal physician who was Professor of Institutes of Medicine at McGill, from 1873–1875, when he was forced to resign because of poor health. Osler took over his lectures in 1874. Drake's name was memorialized later in the Chair of Physiology.

Dreschfeld, Julius (1845–1907. M D, Würzburg; F.R.C.P. Professor of Pathology, later of Medicine, Victoria University, Manchester, England.

Eaton, Sir John C. (1876–1922). He was the son of the founder of T. Eaton Co., Ltd. (department stores). He lived in Toronto and became president of the company. Among his civic interests, he was a member of the Board of Trustees of the Toronto General Hospital and the University of Toronto.

Eberts, Beatrice Muriel (Mrs. E.M.) (1875–1913). Daughter of R.P. and Emily Howard, sister of Campbell. Married August 24, 1904. Osler was devoted to her from her earliest years. Died suddenly in puerperium from phlebitis. Mother of Hermann L. (1905–1982); Edmond H. (1906–1977); Beatrice E. (Mrs. C.E. Price), (1908–   ): Adelaide F. (Mrs. C.P. Cooley), (1910–   ): and Christopher C. (1913–1975).

Eberts, Edmond Melchior (1873–1946). M D, McGill, 1897. Married B. Muriel Howard. Surgeon to Montreal General Hospital; Professor of Surgery at McGill University.

Edes, Robert T. (1838–1923). M D, Harvard, 1861. Taught materia medica at Harvard until he became Professor of Clinical Medicine, 1884–1886. One of the founders of Association of

American Physicians, 1885. After five years of practice in Washington, D.C., he returned to consulting practice in neurological disorders in Boston, 1891–1915.

Edward, Prince of Wales (1894–1972). Eldest son of King George V. On Army Staff during World War I, and travelled widely while Prince of Wales. He became King Edward VIII in January 1936, but abdicated in December of that year. Later, he served the Commonwealth as Duke of Windsor.

Edwards, Arthur R. (1867–1936). M D, Chicago Medical College, 1891. Professor of Principles and Practice of Medicine and Clinical Medicine, Northwestern University, 1892–1917, and later, Dean of Medicine. Wrote a textbook on the practice of medicine.

Ehrlich, Paul (1854–1915). M D, Berlin. During his career he devised staining techniques for white blood cells and the tubercle bacillus. He studied the chemical reactions of cells to oxygen, dyes and other chemicals. His side-chain theory of chemical receptors aided his researches on serum therapy, and later, his discoveries of treatments for trypanosomal and spirochetal diseases. Assisted by S. Hata, Ehrlich introduced the arsenical treatment for syphilis (1910–12). Osler and A. G. Gibson visited Ehrlich's laboratory at Frankfurt in 1907.

Eiselberg, Anton von (1860–1939). Pupil of Billroth and became Professor of Surgery at Vienna in 1901. First to report tetany following total removal of parathyroids during thyroidectomy, 1890.

Elvehjem, Conrad A. (1901–1962). Ph D, Wisconsin, 1927. In Department of Biochemistry from 1927, professor, 1936–58, and Chairman, 1944–58. He was Dean of the Graduate School, 1946–58, and then, President, University of Wisconsin. Elvehjem devoted his career to animal nutrition. In 1937, his group proved nicotinic acid cured canine black-tongue. They established that nicotinic acid was in active liver extracts, and they continued to identify and describe new vitamins. Elvehjem received many national scientific honors.

Emerson, Charles P. (1872–1938). MD, Johns Hopkins, 1899. House Officer, Assistant Resident and Resident Physician under Osler and L.F. Barker, Johns Hopkins Hospital, 1899–1908. Assistant Professor of Medicine Cornell University, 1909–10; Professor of Medicine and Dean, University of Indiana, Indianapolis, 1911–32, and research professor after 1932. President of the Association of American Medical Colleges; Co-author of *Physiology and Hygiene,* and author of several books on clinical medicine and hospitals.

Emmons, Robert Van B. (c. 1895–   ). An Oxford undergraduate who shared his friend Revere's interest in books. During Revere's leave from military duty, the friends usually met in Oxford. William Osler is pictured with Emmons as an undergraduate (Cushing, *Life,* II, p. 378).

Enoch, W.H. (c. 1892–   ). First employed at the Bodleian Library in July 1912; soon appointed a minor assistant in the catalogue revision section. Thence Osler's librarian-secretary from August, 1913, until he entered military service during June, 1915.

Ewald, Carl Anton (1845–1915). M D, Berlin, 1870. Berlin professor and authority on stomach disorders who introduced the gastric test-meal. Osler and Ewald were on the 1903 program of the Association of American Physicians.

Favill, Henry Baird (1860–1916). M D, Rush, 1883. Professor of Clinical Medicine, Rush Medical College, Chicago.

Finley, Frederick G. (1861–1940). M D, McGill, 1885; LL D, McGill. Interned at the Montreal General Hospital. He began teaching in 1889, and was Professor of Medicine, McGill, and a Senior Physician, Montreal General Hospital, 1907–24. He continued as consultant at Montreal General Hospital and other McGill Hospitals thereafter. Served with Canadian Army in England and France, 1914–18, attaining the rank of Colonel and Consultant in Medicine to the Canadian hospitals in Europe. A student of R.P. Howard and W. Osler, Finley was ever a warm friend of Campbell Howard.

Fitz, Reginald Heber (1843–1913). M D, Harvard, 1868; LL D, Harvard, 1905. He studied with Rokitansky and Skoda in Vienna, Corneil in Paris, and Rudolf Virchow in Berlin. He introduced cellular pathology into America in 1870. Lecturer at Harvard from 1870, becoming Professor of Pathological Anatomy, 1879–1892, and then Professor of the Theory and Practice of Medicine, 1892–1908. Influential on important committees on medical courses at Harvard Medical School. His fame rests on original papers on "Perforating Inflammation of the Vermiform Appendix" (1886), and "Acute Pancreatitis" (1889).

Fitz, Reginald (1885–1953). M D, Harvard, 1909; LL D. Trained in Boston, Baltimore, and New York; then a fellow in physiology at Harvard 1914–15 before joining the U.S. Army Medical Corps in France with No. 5 Base Hospital, attaining the rank of Major. During the war, he met and married Phoebe Wright. From 1920–22, he was on the medical staff of the Mayo Clinic, Rochester Minnesota. At Harvard he was associate professor of Medicine, 1922–36; lecturer in History of Medicine, 1936–53, and assistant Dean of Medicine, 1947–53. Also he was Wade Professor of Medicine, Boston University, 1936–40; Chairman of the Selective Service Medical Advisory Board in Boston, 1940–47; President of the American College of Physicians, 1949–50.

Fletcher, Robert (1823–1912). Qualified in medicine at Bristol and London Hospital, 1844; settled in Cincinnati. He remained in the U.S. government service after the Civil War and joined Billings at Surgeon-General's Library in 1876. Fletcher's role in indexing the *Catalogue* and the *Index Medicus* was recognized by his colleagues and users including W. Osler and H. Cushing. Fletcher was editor-in-chief of *Index Medicus* from 1903–1912.

Flexner, Abraham (1866–1959). A B, Johns Hopkins, 1886, then taught school in Louisville, Kentucky. Ed. D., Harvard, 1906. After further study in Germany, he wrote an analysis of American college education, 1908. He then joined the Carnegie Foundation for the Advancement of Teaching and began a survey of all medical schools in the United States and Canada. Subsequently, he also served on the General Education Board to advise J. D. Rockefeller, and in 1930 he founded and directed the Princeton Institute for Advanced Study. He was a brother of Simon Flexner, M.D. and admiring friend of W. H. Welch. A. Flexner's major works on medical education include: *Medical Education in the United States and Canada: A Report to the Carnegie Foundation . . .*, (New York, 1910), and *Medical Education: A Comparative Study,* (New York, 1925).

Flexner, Simon (1863–1946). M D, Louisville, 1889. Pupil and assistant of W. H. Welch at Johns Hopkins, 1891–98. Then Professor of Pathology at University of Pennsylvania. Director of Rockefeller Institute for Medical Research, 1903–35. Original contributions on cerebrospinal meningitis, poliomyelitis, venoms and epidemiology.

Fox, T. Colcott (1849–1916). M B, London, 1876; F R C P, London, 1892. Physician for skin diseases, Westminster Hospital, London. With his father, Tilbury Fox, he wrote *Epitome of Skin Diseases* (1876), and made many later contributions as well.

Francis, Marian (1841–1915). Daughter of W. Osler's uncle Edward Osler, physician of Swansea and Cornwall. She was the mother of William W. Francis, M.D.

Francis, William Willoughby (1878–1959). M D, Johns Hopkins, 1902. Son of William Osler's cousin, Marian, and grandson of his uncle Edward Osler, physician of Cornwall. He interned at Royal Victoria Hospital, Montreal, 1902–04, and was a Fellow under W. H. Welch in Pathology at Johns Hopkins, 1904–05. After a year studying in Europe, he practiced medicine in Montreal and assisted in Pathology at McGill from 1907–11. Then he required sanitarium care for pulmonary tuberculosis. From 1912–15 he was employed by the Canadian Medical Association, and was assistant editor of its *Journal*. He had read proofs of several editions of Osler's textbook since 1905. He served in France with No. 3 Canadian General Hospital, 1915–19, and after demobilization returned to Oxford during Osler's final illness. He edited the *International Journal of Public Health* in Geneva, 1920–22. He spent the years from 1922–29 at Oxford as the principal editor of the catalogue of William Osler's medical library. His meticulous care for details contributed greatly to the scholarship of the *Bibliotheca Osleriana*. From May 29, 1929, to his death, Francis was curator of the Osler Library in the McGill Medical Building, and interpreted the collection and the life of Sir William Osler with devotion.

Futcher, Thomas Barnes (1871–1938). M D, Toronto, 1893. Married Gwendolen Marjorie Howard, 1909. He was a House Officer, Toronto General Hospital, 1893–94; Assistant Resident, 1894–98, and Resident on Osler's medical service, Johns Hopkins Hospital, 1898–1901. He practiced in Baltimore until his death. He worked in the dispensary and taught clinical medicine, for which he attained the rank of Associate Professor of Medicine. He served as Lieutenant Colonel in charge of medical service at No. 18 Canadian General Hospital in England, 1917–18. Futcher contributed to the literature, and was President of the Association of American Physicians, 1932.

Garrett, John Work (1872–c. 1942). B S, Princeton, 1895. Son of T. Harrison Garrett of Baltimore. His early diplomatic positions were Secretary of American Legation at the Hague, 1901–1903; to the Netherlands and Luxemburg, 1903–05, and to the American Embassy at Berlin, 1906–08. Later, he was stationed at the Embassy in Paris, and signed a treaty in November 1918 regarding prisoners of war in Germany. He was a trustee of Johns Hopkins University, 1937–42.

Garrett, Miss Mary Elizabeth (1854–1915). The daughter of John W. Garrett, one of the original Johns Hopkins University trustees, Miss Garrett had inherited her father's fortune and business interests. Influenced by M. Carey Thomas, she was increasingly interested in women's education. Miss Garrett played an important role in the Women's Fund Committee to raise adequate funds to open the College of Medicine, and late in 1892 she donated over $350,000 of the required $500,000. The Board of Trustees accepted certain of the donor's provisions, of which the most significant was that men and women students be admitted on the same terms. Miss Garrett gave generously to the Medical School later during her life, and by her will.

Garrison, Fielding H. (1870–1935). M D, Georgetown, 1893. He worked as assistant librarian in the Surgeon-General's Library, 1899–1922. He was co-editor of *The Index Medicus,* 1903–12 and editor, 1912–27. He retired as Colonel in the U.S. Army in 1930, and was then appointed librarian, Welch Medical Library and lecturer on history of medicine, Johns Hopkins Medical School. He was President of the American Association for the History of Medicine. Among his works are *An Introduction to the History of Medicine,* (Philadelphia: W. B. Saunders, 1913; 4th edition, 1929), and "History of Neurology" in Charles L. Dana: *Textbook of Nervous Diseases* (1925). The neurology history was revised as a book by L. C. McHenry, Jr. (Springfield, Illinois: Charles C Thomas, 1969).

Garrod, Archibald E. (1857–1936). M B, Oxford, 1884 and M D, 1886, F R C P, 1891; LL D, Glasgow and others. F. R. S., 1910. Trained at Christ Church, Oxford and St. Bartholomew's Hospital, London; attended and promoted full physician at St. Bartholomew's Hospital. Regius Professor of Medicine, Oxford, 1920–27. In addition to *Inborn Errors of Metabolism*

(1909), he wrote *Inborn Factors of Disease,* (1931), and many notable addresses.

Gates, Frederick T. (1853–1929). M A, University of Rochester, 1879; graduate Rochester Theology Seminar, 1880. LL D, Chicago, 1911. Baptist Minister who was engaged as business and benevolent representative of John D. Rockefeller, 1893–1912. Chariman of Trustees, Rockefeller Institute for Medical Research; director of Rockefeller Foundation, General Education Board, etc.

Gaylord, Harvey R. (1872–1924). M D, Pennsylvania, 1893. Trained in pathology in Philadelphia during Osler's tenure, he later practiced pathology and bacteriology in Buffalo, N.Y.

Geddes, Lord Auckland (1879–1954). M B, 1903; M D, Edinburgh, 1908. He held appointments in anatomy at Edinburgh and in Ireland before occupying the Chair of Anatomy, McGill University in 1913. He then served with the Royal Army Medical Corps, 1914–16, before joining Lloyd George's administration as Director of Recruiting. He also held several cabinet posts. He accepted the offer to be Principal of McGill to take effect in 1920, but resigned when appointed British Ambassador to the United States, 1920–24. After a career in business, he rejoined government service in 1939, as World War II was imminent. He was made a Knight in 1917, and raised to the Peerage in 1942.

Gesner, Conrad (1516–1565). A Swiss naturalist, appointed Professor of Natural History at Zurich in 1555. A prolific writer, he is famous for books on botany and zoology, but above all as the earliest great bibliographer. For his 20 volume *Bibliotheca Universalis* (1545–49), Osler placed Gesner in the *prima* section of the *Bibliotheca Osleriana.*

Gibson, Alexander, G. (1875–1950). M B, 1904; M D, Oxford, 1908. F.R.C.P., London. Served as house officer at Radcliffe Infirmary, Oxford from 1904; then pathologist from 1911, and was

senior physician 1919–44. He assisted Osler in editing the
Quarterly Journal of Medicine in 1907, and later he joined
the Editorial Board. Wrote *The Radcliffe Infirmary* (1926),
and several works on internal medicine, including an early
clinical and pathological account of ischemic heart disease.

Gibson, George A. (1854–1913). M B, 1876, and M D, D Sc., Edinburgh. LL D, McGill and others. He was a resident physician, on the honorary attending staff, and later Physician to
the Royal Infirmary, Edinburgh. He wrote *Diseases of the
Heart and Aorta* (1898), etc.

Gibson, Robert B. (1882–1959). Ph.D., Yale, 1906. Taught physiological chemistry at Minnesota, Missouri, and Philippines Universities, 1907–1919. He was Assistant Professor of Medicine,
1919–28; Director, Clinical Chemical Laboratory, 1919–50;
Associate Professor of Biochemistry, 1928–50; Professor,
1950–52; Emeritus, 1952–59, State University of Iowa. Gibson's research work with C.P. Howard led to early publications on the effects of diet on metabolism in pernicious
anemia. Later, he continued research on diabetes mellitus,
anemias and other disorders.

Gilman, Daniel Coit (1831–1908), A.M. Yale 1852; LL D, Harvard
and others. Professor of physical and political geography,
Yale, 1856–72. President of University of California, 1872–
75. First President, Johns Hopkins University, 1876–1901.
Served on important U.S. Commissions. Author of several
books, including *University Problems* (1888), *Launching of
a University* (1906). Osler dedicated *Aequanimitas* to Gilman.

Goldberger, Joseph (1874–1929). M D, Bellevue Hospital Medical
College, 1895. Commissioned in U.S. Public Health Service,
1899, he contributed to knowledge of several infectious diseases. From 1913, he studied pellagra and demonstrated
that its cause was a deficiency of a pellagra-preventive factor. He died before niacin was identified.

Goodnow, Frank J. (1859–1939). Political scientist and educator. M A, Amherst, 1887; LL D, Amherst and others. Teacher at Columbia, 1883–1907. President of Johns Hopkins University, 1914–29. Author of books on political science and constitutional law.

Gordon, Alvah H. (1876–1953). M D, McGill, 1899. LL D, McGill and others. Interned at Montreal General Hospital; practiced in British Columbia until 1902, when he returned to the Montreal General Hospital and McGill; Associate Professor, 1924–1936, then Professor and Chairman of Medicine at the Montreal General Hospital, 1936–39. President, American Clinical and Climatological Association, 1939, and of the Association of American Physicians, 1948.

Graham, Duncan A. (1882–1974), M B, Toronto, 1905. LL D, F.R.C.P. (London). Trained in bacteriology and pathology at the Toronto General Hospital, in the United States and abroad prior to appointment as lecturer in bacteriology, Toronto, 1911–15. Served in World War I with No. 4 Canadian General Hospital in Salonika, attaining the rank of Lieutenant Colonel. He was then appointed John Eaton Professor and Chairman of Medicine, University of Toronto, and Physician in Chief, Toronto General Hospital, 1919–47. He was president of the Royal College of Physicians (Canada), 1933–1935, the Canadian Medical Association, 1940, and an honored member of other Societies and Research Committees. He trained many pupils, including several professors of medicine at Canadian Universities.

Graham, Willard T. (1863–1932). M D, Medical College of Ohio, 1886. He left the administration of Methodist Hospital, Des Moines, to serve as Superintendant of University of Iowa Hospitals, Iowa City, from January 1916–1921. After an interval in New York State, he returned in poor health to the Superintendant's staff in Iowa City. He served as host at the University Hospital from 1928 until he suffered a fatal stroke in April, 1932.

Graves, Robert James (1797–1853). M B, Trinity, Dublin, 1818. Wrote clear "Clinical Lectures" based on pathological studies at Meath Hospital. Professor of Institutes of Medicine at Trinity College, Dublin, 1827–41. Leader of famous "Irish school" with colleagues, W. Stokes and R. Townsend. Graves' name is attached to exophthalmic goiter.

Gross, Samuel D. (1805–1884). M D, Jefferson, 1828. After practicing in Cincinnati, and being Professor of Surgery at Louisville, 1840–56, he returned to the Chair at Jefferson Medical College, Philadelphia. His operative skills and publications on genitourinary diseases, experimental surgery, and a two-volume system of surgery brought him fame. He also wrote biographies of surgeons and histories of American surgery.

Gross, Samuel W. (1837–1889) M.D. Jefferson Medical College, 1857. Son of Samuel D. Gross. Married Grace Linzee Revere, December, 1876. Professor of Surgery, Jefferson Medical College, 1882. Wrote on military surgery, malignant growths, and male sexual disorders.

Guthrie, James R. (1858–1930). M D, Iowa, 1884. Resided and practiced in Dubuque, Iowa, 1885–1930. Professor of Physiology, 1889–1902; Professor of Obstetrics and Gynecology, 1898–1915, and Dean of Medicine, 1902–14, University of Iowa. President of Iowa State Medical Society, 1901–02, and of the Association of American Medical Colleges, 1903–04.

Gwyn, Major C. Campbell (1884–1917). Son of Colonel Gwyn and William Osler's sister, Charlotte. He served with the Canadian Infantry in France from 1914 until 1917 when he was killed.

Gwyn, E.H. Nona (Mrs. Cecil Stuart) (1889–1965). Daughter of William Osler's sister, Charlotte. She was a close friend of Ottilie Wright.

Gwyn, Norman B. (1875–1952). M B, Toronto, 1896. Son of William Osler's sister, Charlotte. He was assistant resident physician, Johns Hopkins Hospital, 1898–1900, and practiced in Philadelphia. During World War I, he served in the Canadian Army Medical Corps overseas where his final appointment was Lieutenant Colonel in charge of the medical service, No. 1 Canadian General Hospital. Following the war, he practiced in Toronto at the Toronto General and Christie Street Hospitals, and helped arrange the Osler and other collections at the Academy of Medicine. He contributed several articles about Osler.

Haldane, John S. (1860–1936). MD Edinburgh (1884). D.Sc. Oxford. L L D Edinburgh and Birmingham. Fellow of Royal Society. Conducted investigations in physiology and chemistry at Oxford beginning 1887 and continuing throughout his career. Consultant to British Services in World War I. Made original contributions to oxygen, carbon dioxide and hemoglobin determinations (1892–1901), the administration of oxygen by mask (1917), and others.

Hale-White, Sir William (1857–1949). M D, London, LL D, Edinburgh. Trained at Guy's Hospital, 1875; Physician to Guy's Hospital, 1890–1919. Knighted in 1919. Wrote *Materia Medica, Pharmacy, Pharmacology and Therapeutics* (1892; ed. 27, 1947); *Common Affections of the Liver* (1908), and many other works.

Halsted, William Stewart (1852–1922). M D, College of Physicians and Surgeons, New York, 1877. Trained in Vienna and German clinics, 1878–80. Operated and taught at the College of Physicians and Surgeons with distinction, 1880–85. Experiments led to introduction of block anesthesia with cocaine, 1885. After surgical research with Welch and Mall at Johns Hopkins, he became the first surgeon of the Johns Hopkins Hospital, 1889, and Professor of Surgery, 1892– 1922. Halsted developed surgical procedures after detailed animal studies. He advanced techniques for cancer of breast, inguinal hernia, and in other areas. He taught me-

ticulous dissection with aseptic technique and control of
all bleeding vessels.

Hamburger, Franz (1874–1954). German physician who introduced a modified tuberculin skin test, and published frequently on tuberculosis in children.

Harvey, William (1578–1657). M B, Cambridge, 1597; M D, Padua,
1602. Physician of London and a prominent Fellow and
supporter of the College of Physicians of London. He is
acknowledged as the greatest English biomedical scientist
before the 19th century. Author of *Exercitatio anatomica de
motu cordis et sanguinis in animalibus* [*On the Movement
of the Heart and Blood in Animals*] (1628), and *Exercita-
tiones de generatione animalium* (1651).

Hektoen, Ludvig (1863–1951) M D, Illinois, 1887, Professor of Pathology and Bacteriology, 1901–51, and also Director of
McCormick Institute of Infectious Diseases, University of
Chicago, 1902–37. Conducted significant research on im-
munology. Editor *Journal of Infectious Diseases* and *Archives of Pathology*. Twice Chairman of Medical Division
of National Research Council.

Herrick James B. (1861–1954). MD, Rush, 1888. Trained and practiced at Cook County Hospital, Chicago, and Professor of
Clinical Medicine, University of Illinois. Wrote "Clinical
Features of Sudden Obstruction of the Coronary Arteries"
(1912), and additional work of fundamental importance in
the understanding of coronary thrombosis. He also contributed on sickle cell anemia, and was recognized a leader
of medicine in Chicago and America.

Hewetson, John (1867–1910). M D, McGill, 1891. Interned at Montreal General Hospital; Assistant resident on Osler's medical
service, Johns Hopkins Hospital, 1891–94. While studying in
Leipzig, Germany, during the winter of 1895, acute manifestations of pulmonary tuberculosis appeared, which pro-

gressed and finally caused his death. Osler wrote a heart-rending memorial in *Bulletin of Johns Hopkins Hospital* 21 (December 1910), p. 357.

Hewlett, Albion Walter (1874–1925). M D, Johns Hopkins, 1900. Director of the clinical laboratory, University of Michigan, 1908–1916, and later also Professor of Medicine. In 1916, he became Professor of Medicine, Leland Stanford Junior School of Medicine.

Horsley, Sir Victor (1857–1916). Qualified 1881. F.R.S., F.R.C.S., Knighted in 1902. He trained at University College and Hospital, London, and joined the surgical staff in 1885; Professor of Pathology, 1887–96; Professor of Clinical Surgery, 1889–1915. He participated in laboratory research through 1913. In World War I, he embarked for Egypt in 1915, and was a Colonel performing field surgery in Mesopotamia when he died from heat stroke. His publications included the use of thyroid gland to treat myxedema, the electrical method of localization in the nervous system, and surgical treatment of intracranial tumors. Osler contributed a personal note to his obituary (*British Medical Journal,* July 29, 1916).

Howard, Sir Arthur Jared P. (1896–1971). Knighted in 1953. Younger son of R. Jared B. Howard. He served in World War I with Scots Guards, 1914–17; retired as Captain because of severe wounds; Croix de Guerre. Principal Warden, London Civil Defense Region, 1939–42. M P, 1945–50. Treasurer, St. George's Hospital, 1943–64.

Howard, Robert Henry P. (Harry) (1893–1915). Second son of Campbell's brother, Jared. While a subaltern with the Royal East Surrey Regiment at the Battle of Ypres, he was killed on May 9, 1915.

Howard, R. Jared B. (1859–1921). M D, McGill, 1882. F.R.C.S. (England). Studied in London and Germany; then was pathologist and assistant surgeon at the Montreal General Hospital; demonstrator in anatomy and surgery, McGill, and practiced with his father. He married in 1888 and moved to London in the early 1890's. During World War I, he organized a hospital for officers, and worked actively at the 3rd London General Hospital at Wandsworth.

Howard, Hon. Mrs. R.J.B. (Miss Margaret Charlotte Smith) (1854–1926). She was born in Canada as the only child of Mr. and Mrs. Donald Smith, who later became Lord and Lady Strathcona and Mount Royal. By a special provision, she succeeded to the Barony on her father's death in 1914. Her eldest son, Donald, succeeded her, and Arthur and two daughters also survived her.

Howland, John (1873–1926). M D, New York University, 1897. Trained also in Berlin and Vienna. A pupil of Emmett Holt, Howland became head of Children's Clinic at Bellevue Hospital in 1908. In 1912, he succeeded von Pirquet as Professor of Pediatrics at Johns Hopkins Medical School. Among his important research were studies on rickets, and the metabolism of calcium and phosphorus.

Hughes, Lt. Gen. Sir Sam (1853–1921). Member of Canadian Parliament from 1892–1916; Minister of Militia and Defense of Canada, 1911–16.

Humpton, Blanche O. (c. 1869–c.1943). Osler's secretary from the writing of his textbook in 1891, through his tenure at Johns Hopkins, and she maintained a professional and personal correspondence with him until his death. She had continued with L.F. Barker, and assumed responsibility for his private practice office until her retirement.

Hurd, Henry Mills (1843–1927). MD, Michigan (1866) Superintendant of Eastern Michigan Hospital for the Insane, Pontiac, Mich. (1878–1889); Superintendant of Johns Hospital Hospital (1889–1911), and then Secretary of the Board of Trustees of the Hospital.

Hutchinson, Sir Jonathan (1828–1913). Qualified in 1850. After training in various London institutions, he became Senior Surgeon at the London Hospital, 1873–83. FRS, 1882. Fellow of the Royal College of Surgeons and President, 1889. He taught at the Medical Graduates' College and Polyclinic, and contributed to its museum. Osler frequently praised Hutchinson for his general contributions to the medical profession, and the large museum at his home in Haslemere. Hutchinson described the typical deformities of the teeth in congenital syphilis, and also wrote many articles on surgery, ophthalmology, dermatology and neurology.

Jacobi, Abraham (1830–1919). M D, Bonn, Germany, 1851; came to New York City in 1854 to practice, with special interest in children's diseases. In 1860, he became the first professor of pediatrics in New York City, for most years at College of Physicians and Surgeons of New York, 1870–1899. President of the American Pediatric Society, the Association of American Physicians and others. Wrote important articles, and was recognized as the leading American pediatrician.

Jacobi, Mary Putnam (1842–1906). After graduating in Pharmacy, she achieved the M.D. from Woman's Medical College of Pennsylvania, 1864 and L'École de Médecine, Paris, 1871. Then she taught at the Woman's Medical College of New York Infirmary, became a member of the County Medical Society and married Abraham Jacobi. She contributed articles of high literary quality to the medical literature, especially on pediatrics and neurology.

Jacobs, Henry Barton (1858–1939). MD, Harvard, 1887. Attended the dispensary in medicine, Johns Hopkins Hospital, 1896–1904. Secretary and a director of the National Tuberculosis Association, 1904–20, and affiliated with tuberculosis institutions in Maryland while practicing in Baltimore. A Trustee of Johns Hopkins Hospital, 1911–39, the Harriet Lane Home for Children and other institutions. He was given a latchkey to Osler's house in Baltimore, and continued a close friendship thereafter.

Janeway, Theodore Caldwell (1872–1917). M D, Columbia, 1895. After other affiliations in New York City, he joined the faculty of Columbia University in 1907, and became Professor of Medicine, 1909–1914. In 1914, under the William Welch Endowment, Janeway accepted a full-time position as Chairman of Medicine, Johns Hopkins University, a post he held until his death. He combined physiology and pathology with clinical medicine. He was engaged also in military duties in Baltimore and Washington from April 1917 until death from pneumonia, December 27, 1917. Published "Clinical Study of Blood Pressure" (1904). A detailed manuscript on diseases of the heart and blood vessels was nearing completion at his death.

Jelliffe, Smith Ely (1866–1945). MD, College of Physicians and Surgeons, New York (1886). Prominent New York neurologist and psychiatrist. Editor of *The Medical News* (New York, 1900–08), and later the *Psychoanalytic Review,* and the Nervous and Mental Disease Monograph Series. He wrote many articles including Chapters on "Hysteria" and "Migraine" for Osler and McCrae's *System of Medicine* (Oxford, 1910).

Jepson, William (1863–1945). M D, Iowa 1886; M D, Pennsylvania, 1891. Began practice in Sioux City, 1892. Postgraduate training in Edinburgh, 1897. Professor of Surgery, Sioux City College of Medicine, 1891–1901; Professor and Chairman of Surgery, State University of Iowa, 1902–1912. He spent two days in Iowa City and remainder of week in Sioux City. In 1911, he considered residing in Iowa City, but late in 1912 he resigned his professorship to continue his surgical practice in Sioux City. He was President of the Iowa State Medical Society, 1905–06; Fellow of American College of Surgeons.

He served on active duty with U.S. Army Medical Corps, 1916–18.

Jessup, Walter A. (1877–1944). A B, Earlham, 1903; Ph.D, Columbia, 1911. Dean, College of Education, State University of Iowa, 1913–16, and President, 1916–34. He was President of the Carnegie Foundation for the Advancement of Teaching, 1934–44, and President, Carnegie Corporation, New York, 1941–44.

Johnson, Rev. William A. (1816–1880). Born in Bombay to a British military family, his early life was spent in England until he migrated to Canada in 1831. In 1851, he was ordained in the Toronto diocese of the Anglican church. He held the high church beliefs of the minority of his colleagues and parishioners. Near Weston (now within the city of Toronto) he started a private school for boys in the early 1860's. This became a preparatory school in association with Trinity College in 1864 with Johnson as Warden. He inspired many boys to share his interest in natural history by teaching them the collection of specimens, and preparation and examination of microscopic slides. Johnson's friendship with William Osler was strained only by apprehension that his pupil veer from his own strict theology.

Jones, Surgeon-General Guy Carleton (1864–1950). Qualified in England, 1887; licensed in Nova Scotia in 1890; entered the Canadian Army Medical Corps before World War I. He was Director General of the Canadian Medical Services in Europe, 1914–16, and later in Canada. He retired in 1920.

Kelly, Howard A. (1858–1943). M D, Pennsylvania, 1882. Professor of gynecology, University of Pennsylvania (1888), and the first Professor of Gynecology at Johns Hopkins (1889–1919). Established long-term residency training in gynecology. Through his pupils, his innovative operating techniques and his talented methods of education by demonstrations,

stereo-optic photographs and publications, he attained a
leading position in gynecology. He contributed to medical
history and biography, and participated actively in religion
and philosophy. He was a friend of William Osler.

Kenyon, Sir Frederic George (1863–1952). Classics degrees at New
College, Oxford in 1883, 1886. He worked in the manus-
cripts department at the British Museum from 1888, and
was director of the Museum, 1909–30. He published articles
and books on topics ranging from Greek papyri to the
Brownings.

Kerr, James (1848–1911). M D, Queens', Belfast, 1870. Surgeon to
mines near Londonderry, N.S., Canada from 1874–80. He
was a pioneer of Listerian surgery in Canada, and became
a friend of F.J. Shepherd and William Osler. On July 26,
1876, Kerr married a first cousin of A. Graham Bell in Brantford, Ont. Osler was his best man. After 1880, Kerr practiced and taught surgery in Montreal, Winnipeg and Washington, D.C., where he retired in 1907.

Keynes, Sir Geoffrey (1887–1982). M D, Cambridge, LL D.,
F.R.C.P., F.R.C.S. (England, Canada), F.R.C.O.G.; knighted
in 1955. Trained at St. Bartholomew's Hospital, 1913. Served
in R.A.M.C., 1914–19. On Surgical staff of Bartholomew's
Hospital from 1920. He wrote *Blood Transfusion* (1922,
1949) and many professional articles; bibliographies of Sir
Thomas Browne (in which he acknowledged Osler's inspiration), William Harvey, Robert Hooke, William Blake, Jane
Austen and others. Edited letters of William Blake; and
wrote biographies of Blake, Harvey and many others. Ap-
pended to his autobiography, *The Gates of Memory* (1981)
is a reprint of his article, "The Oslerian Tradition".

Kipling, Rudyard (1865–1936). British author born in India, he was
familiar with Anglo-Indian life. He was famous for short
stories, poems, and novels. Often he extolled the British
Empire as it existed before World War I.

Klebs, Arnold C. (1870–1943). M D, Basel, 1895. He lived in the
United States and worked chiefly in Chicago between 1896–
1909. He directed the Chicago Tuberculosis Institute, and
assisted the National Tuberculosis Association. Klebs returned to Europe, but frequently returned to the United
States visits of varying durations. An ardent bibliophile and
scholar, Klebs collaborated with Harvey Cushing and John
Fulton in donating the books to start the History of Medicine Library at Yale University in 1939.

Klotz, Oskar (1878–1936). M B, Toronto, 1902. M D, McGill, 1906.
He trained at McGill, the Rockefeller Foundation and Universities of Bonn and Freiburg through 1908, and Marburg
in 1914. He also had junior appointments in pathology at
McGill from 1905–09. He was Professor of Pathology, University of Pittsburg, 1909–20, at Sao Paulo, Brazil, 1921–23,
and at the University of Toronto, 1923–36. He was president
of the American Association of Pathologists and Bacteriologists, 1919, and the Association of Medical Museums, 1919.

Koch, Robert (1843–1910). M D, Göttingen, 1866. Pupil of Jakob
Henle. While a country practitioner, Koch discovered the
spore-bearing bacillus of anthrax, 1876, and identified several microorganisms capable of cuasing wound infections,
1878. While working in a national laboratory in Berlin, he
identified the tubercle bacillus, 1882, and the cholera vibrio,
1883. In 1885, he became Professor of Hygiene and bacteriology at Berlin; in 1891, Director of his own Institute, and in
1905 was awarded the Nobel Prize.

Kraeplin, Emil (1856–1926). Famous German psychiatrist. After
1904, Chief, Münchner Kreisirrenanstals Psychiatrist Klinik,
Munich.

Kraus, Friedrich (1858–1936). M D, Prague, 1882. First engaged in
chemistry and pathology; then in clinical medicine in Graz
and Vienna. From 1902, he was in the II University Clinic
at Charity Hospital, Berlin. He participated in Osler's sec-

tion at the International Medical Congress in London, 1913. He wrote on various pathophysiological and clinical subjects. He emphasized the study of the patient as a whole person.

Krehl, Ludolf von (1861–1937). Professor at Strasburg prior to transfer to Heidelberg in 1906. He approached clinical problems from the patho-physiological view.

Laënnec, René T.A. (1781–1826). A native of Brittany, he studied medicine in Paris under Corvisart and Bichat, and rapidly gained prominence as a clinician. He introduced the stethoscope for the diagnosis of disorders of the heart and lungs (1819).

Lafleur, Henri A. (1862–1939). MD, McGill (1887). House physician and pathologist, Montreal General Hospital, 1886–89. First resident of Osler at Johns Hopkins Hospital, 1889–91. Then returned to McGill and Montreal General Hospital at which he became Professor of Medicine and Clinical Medicine at McGill, and Physician to the Hospital, 1907–1921. An excellent lecturer, Lafleur was also an outstanding clinician, following the ways of Osler.

Laveran, Charles L.A. (1845–1922), French Army Surgeon famous for the discovery of malaria parasites in human red blood cells. He was awarded the Nobel Prize in 1907.

Leidy, Joseph (1823–1891). M D, Pennsylvania, 1844. He practiced for two years and taught anatomy for a year before he joined Professor Horner's Department at Pennsylvania in 1847. Leidy was Professor of Anatomy, Pennsylvania, 1858–1891. He made original contributions to several aspects of medical science including comparative anatomy. Osler greatly admired his senior colleague at Philadelphia. Among his most famous works was *Fresh Water Rhizopods of North America* (1879).

Lewis, Sir Thomas (1881–1945). M B, M D, London, 1904, 1907; FRCP, 1913; Fellow Royal Society, 1918. Director of the Department of Clinical Research and Physician to University College Hospital, London. With A.S. MacNalty, first used the electrocardiograph in humans (1908). He introduced the term auricular fibrillation (1909), and defined variations in the origin of the galvanic impulse (1910–11). Lewis edited *Clinical Science*. His published books included *The Mechanism of the Heart Beat* (1911); *The Soldier's Heart and the Effort Syndrome* (1919) and *The Blood Vessels of the Human Skin and Their Responses* (1927).

Linacre, Thomas (c. 1460–1524). M D, Padua and Oxford. Trained in Italy during the Renaissance, he returned to practice in London. In 1518, he was a founder and first president of the "College Perpetual" in London, the forerunner of the Royal College of Physicians. Osler admired him especially for his excellent Latin translations from Galen's Greek medical treatises.

Little, Herbert M. (Butch) (1877–1934). M D, McGill, 1901. Assistant, 1901–04, and Resident Obstetrician, Johns Hopkins Hospital, 1904–05. Member of the McGill Medical Faculty (from 1907); later, Professor of Obstetrics at McGill, and Gynecologist at the Montreal General Hospital. Fellow of the American College of Surgeons, Royal College of Surgeons (Canada), and College of Obstetricians and Gynecologists (England). Vice-president of the American Association of Obstetricians and Gynecologists.

Lloyd George, David (1863–1945) British Liberal politician; Prime Minister 1916–1922. Credited with raising British morale during World War I, especially towards the end, in 1917–1918.

Locke, John (1632–1704). A Puritan adherent, Locke received the B.A. and M.A. degrees at Oxford by 1658. Influenced by Robert Boyle in science and his friend, Sydenham, in clinical medicine, Locke took the M B degree in 1674. He wrote medical essays and case reports from his prolonged, though intermittent, practice. He spent many years as adviser to Lord Ashley, the chief founder of the Carolina Colony. Locke is credited with writing the Constitution of the Colony, which later served as the model for the Constitution of the United States. Among Locke's philosophical writings is the famous, *Essay Concerning Humane Understanding* (1690). Osler published "An Address on John Locke as a Physician" (1900). Osler included Locke in the *prima* section of the *Bibliotheca Osleriana* because of his influence on social and philosophical thought.

Louis, Pierre C.A. (1787–1872). Physician of Paris who studied series of cases thoroughly, and provided classical descriptions of typhoid fever and pulmonary tuberculosis. He introduced the statistical method to compare the effects of two treatments. The inspiration of his teachings was attested to by his pupils from the United States and other nations.

Ludwig, Carl F. W. (1816–1895). M D, Marburg, 1840. After being Professor of Anatomy at Marburg, 1846–49, he concentrated on physiology, in which he was professor successively at Zurich, Vienna and Leipzig, 1865–95. His important contributions to the research technics and mechanisms of physiology were conducted throughout his career, but especially at his Physiological Institute in Leipzig. As the leading physiologist of the century, he is credited with training more than 200 pupils who continued his teaching over the world.

Macbride, Thomas H. (1848–1934). A B, Monmouth, 1869; Ph D, Lenox College, 1895; LL D. Taught at Lenox College, 1870–78; then at State University of Iowa, becoming Professor of Botany, 1884–1914, President, 1914–16; then President Emeritus. Published books on botany and reports on geology.

MacCallum, John Bruce (c. 1876–1905). M D, Johns Hopkins, 1900. He was regarded as one of the brightest students. During his first post-graduate year in anatomical research under Professor Franklin Mall, MacCallum developed pulmonary tuberculosis, from which he succumbed.

MacCallum, William G. (1874–1944). M D, Johns Hopkins, 1897; LL D, Toronto. House medical officer, 1897, Assistant Resident Pathologist, 1898–1900, then resident pathologist and associate professor to 1909, Johns Hopkins Hospital and Medical School. Professor of Pathology, Columbia University, 1909–17, when he returned to be Chairman of the Department at Johns Hopkins. He was a leader in American pathology in the period following W.H. Welch. Author *Textbook of Pathology* (1916); 7th ed. (1944).

Macdonald, Sir William (1831–1917). Prominent Montreal industrialist in the 19th Century. He generously provided funds for an Agricultural College on a rural campus, the Engineering College building, and other important projects of McGill University.

Mackenzie, Sir James (1853–1925). M D, Edinburgh, 1878. F.R.C.P., London; F.R.S., LL D. After training at the Royal Infirmary of Edinburgh, and briefly in Vienna, he entered general practice at Burnley for twenty-eight years. While practicing, he was the first clinical investigator of cardiac arrhythmias and published "The Study of the Pulse". In 1907, he moved to the London Hospital as physician and lecturer in cardiac research. The next year he published his famous, *Diseases of the Heart*. During World War I, Mackenzie helped to evaluate structural and functional cardiac disorders in soldiers. From 1920–24, he worked at his newly formed Institute for Clinical Research at St. Andrews University. Among later publications were *Principles of Diagnosis and Treatment in Heart Disease* (1916) and *Angina Pectoris* (1924).

MacLean, George E. (1850–1938). Ph D, Leipzig, 1883; LL D, Williams, 1895, and others. Professor of English, Education.

Chancellor, University of Nebraska, 1895–99. President, State University of Iowa, 1899–1911. From 1913, he was a specialist in higher education for the United States Education Commission, assigned to visit Universities and Colleges in Great Britain and Ireland, and then he was appointed Director for Universities and Colleges in United Kingdom, 1918–19; Director of British Division, American Universities Union in Europe, 1919–23. Osler and MacLean helped found the Post-Graduate Medical Association in Great Britain, April, 1919.

MacNalty, Sir Arthur S. (1880–1969). Qualified 1907; M D, 1911; D P H, 1927. F.R.C.P., F.R.C.S. (Eng.). Knighted in 1936. Neurological training under Sir Victor Horsley. Entered government service in 1913, and rose to be Chief Medical Officer, Ministry of Health, 1935–40. Author of *Epidemic Diseases of Central Nervous System* (1927); *History of State Medicine in England* (1948), *The Three Churchills* (1949), and other novels.

Malloch, T. Archibald (1887–1953). M D, McGill, 1913. F.R.C.P. Son of Osler's friend, Dr. A.E. Malloch of Hamilton, Ont., and husband of Katherine E. Abbott, who was a duaghter of Georgina Osler, and thus a granddaughter of William Osler's brother, Featherstone. Served with Red Cross and Canadian Army Medical Corps in Europe, 1914–19. Co-editor of *Bibliotheca Osleriana*. Librarian, New York Academy of Medicine, 1925–53. President, American Library Association, 1927–29.

Manson, Sir Patrick (1844–1922). M D, Aberdeen, 1866. LL D, Aberdeen, 1886, F.R.S., 1900, D Sc., Oxford, 1904. Gained fame for establishing transmission by the mosquito of the filaria of elephantiasis. His work also played a part in establishing the role of mosquitoes in carrying malaria. From 1912, he was Senior Teacher in the London School of Tropical Medicine.

Marburg, William A. (1849–1931). Baltimore philanthropist. He was a Trustee, Johns Hopkins Hospital, 1901–31, and Vice-president of Board of Trustees from 1910. W.A. Marburg donated the Warrington Collection of Books to the Johns Hopkins Medical School, 1907, and contributed to the Charles L. Marburg Memorial Fund, which provided the new private ward building in 1914.

Marie, Pierre (1853–1940). M D, Paris, 1883. Trained by J. M. Charcot, he was a professor in Paris from 1889, and attained the chair of neurology in 1918. Described acromegaly (1886) and hypertophic pulmonary dystrophy (1890). He wrote introduction to Osler's *La Practique de Médecine* (1908).

Martin, Charles F. (1868–1953). M D, McGill, 1892; LLD, Queens, 1927, McGill and Harvard. Trained in Montreal and Germany. Assistant Physician, Royal Victoria Hospital, Montreal, 1895, and promoted to Physician and Professor of Medicine, McGill, 1907–36. Dean of Medicine, McGill, 1923–36, in which position his success has been widely acknowledged. President of the Canadian Medical Association, 1923, of the American College of Physicians, 1929, and of the Association of Medical Colleges. Dean Martin was influential in establishing the Montreal Neurological Institute, and in bringing both J.C. Meakins and C.P. Howard to McGill in 1924 as Professors of Medicine and Physicians-in-Chief at the two large teaching hospitals.

Matthews, Annabel Margaret ("Amo") (1878–1961). Daughter of William Osler's brother, Edmund Boyd Osler, she married Wilmot L. Matthews in 1903.

Max-Müller, Rt. Hon. Friedrich (1823–1900). M A, LL D, DCL. Educated in Universities of Leipzig and Berlin. Professor, Modern Languages, Oxford, 1854–67; and Corpus Professor, Comparative Philology, Oxford, 1868–1900. Publications on Sanskrit literature and the science of language. His widow rented the house at 7 Norham Gardens to the Oslers, 1905–06. Later, her two grandsons were frequent visitors at "The Open Arms". Osler relaxed in the company of the young boys during the stresses of World War I.

Mayo, Charles H. (1865–1939). M D, Northwestern, 1888. Younger son of Dr. William W. Mayo. He was a very able surgeon, and thoughtful colleague and counsellor of his brother, Dr. W.J. Mayo, in the development of the Mayo Clinic.

Mayo, William J. (1861–1939). M D, Michigan, 1883. Elder son of Dr. William W. Mayo (1819–1911), who founded the clinic in 1889 in association with the new St. Mary's Hospital, Rochester, Minn. Dr. W. J. Mayo was an eminent surgeon, and the chief organizer of the famous surgical and multi-disciplinary Mayo Clinic.

McClintock, John T. (1873–1955). M D, Iowa, 1898. Demonstrator in anatomy, University of Iowa, 1898–1901. Trained in physiology under Ludwig and His at Leipzig, 1901–02. Professor of Physiology, Iowa, 1902, until Emeritus rank; also Associate Dean of Medicine. He studied the history of medicine at the University of Iowa, and wrote the chapter "Medical Education in Iowa" in *One Hundred Years of Iowa Medicine* (1951).

McCrae, Amy Marion (Mrs. Thomas) (1878–1941). Duaghter of Osler's sister, Charlotte Gwyn. Married Osler's former resident in 1908.

McCrae, John (1872–1918) M B, Toronto, 1898. Studied under Osler, and others, at Johns Hopkins Hospital for a year until appointed a Fellow at McGill, and Pathologist, Montreal General Hospital. After brief service during the Boer War in South Africa, he returned to clinical medicine at McGill and the Royal Victoria Hospital. From October, 1914, Major McCrae served as Medical Officer in the Canadian Artillery through the crucial Battle of Ypres, April, 1915. This inspired his famous poem, *In Flanders Fields.* From June, 1915, to January, 1918, he was Lieutenant Colonel in charge of medical wards, No. 3 Canadian General Hospital in France. Orders to appoint him consulting physician to the

1st British Army came the day he contracted severe pneumonia. He had contributed articles in pathology and medicine.

McCrae, Thomas (1870–1935). M B, Toronto, 1895, M D, 1903. Married Amy Marion Gwyn, daughter of Osler's sister, Charlotte. Assistant Resident, 1896–1901; Resident Physician, 1901–04 and Associate in Medicine, 1904–12, Johns Hopkins Hospital. Professor of Medicine, Jefferson Medical College, and Physician to Jefferson and Pennsylvania Hospitals, Philadelphia, 1912–35. Fellow, Royal College of Physicians, London. President of Association of American Physicians, 1930. He authored many articles and assisted Osler in revising 8th edition of the *Principles and Practice of Medicine*, 1912; was co-author of 9th edition (1920) and alone revised the 11th (1928) and 12th editions (1930). Osler and McCrae also edited the multi-volume system *Modern Medicine, Its Theory and Practice* (Philadelphia: Lea & Febiger, 1907–10), 2nd edition (1913–15), and McCrae alone edited the 3rd edition (1925–1928).

Meakins, John C. (1882–1959). M D, McGill, 1904. Fellow, Royal College of Physicians, Edinburgh, 1919; Fellow Royal Society 1920. Resident physician, Royal Victoria Hospital Montreal, 1904–06. Trained also at Johns Hopkins, and Presbyterian Hospital, New York, before returning to McGill in 1910 in clinical and experimental medicine. During Army Medical Service, 1914–19, he studied irritable heart syndrome at the British Army Hospital at Hampstead, and also investigated the effects of chemical warfare. He was Professor of Therapeutics, Edinburgh University, 1919–24; Professor and Chairman of Medicine, McGill, and Physician-in-Chief, Royal Victoria Hospital, 1924–47; Dean of Medicine, 1942–47. President of Canadian Medical Association, American College of Physicians, and Royal College of Physicians and Surgeons of Canada. He authored many articles on internal medicine, especially on pulmonary and cardiovascular diseases. *The Practice of Medicine* appeared in six editions from 1926–56.

Meredith, Allen Pickton Osler (1889–1975). Son of Arthur and Isobel (Osler) Meredith. Served for several years in the Canadian Infantry in France, attaining the rank of Major. Married Jean Wright on January 4, 1919, at Oxford.

Meredith, Frances Marion Pauline ("Dinah") (1893–). Sister of
Allen Meredith. After World War I, she married James O'-
Reilly.

Meredith, Isobel Marion (Mrs. Arthur) (1868–1937). Daughter of
Edward L.P. Osler, who was a brother of William Osler.

Milburn, Edward F. (1849–1926). William Osler's boyhood friend
from school at Barrie and Weston. He later lived in Belleville, Ontario. Osler corresponded with him throughout his
life. His letters formed the basis of H. L. Holley: A Contin-
ual Remembrance (Springfield, Il.: Charles C Thomas,
1968).

Mitchell, Silas Weir (1829–1914). M D, Jefferson, 1850; LL D, Harvard, 1886, and others. President, Association of American
Physicians, 1881, and College of Physicians of Philadelphia.
Studied wounds of the nervous system in Civil War. Later
taught at Orthopedic Hospital and Infirmary for Nervous
Diseases, Philadelphia. Introduced rest treatment for neuroses in Fat and Blood (1877), and Lectures on Diseases of
the Nervous System, Especially in Women (1881). He also
presented many original clinical descriptions and addresses, "William Harvey" and "Instruments of Precision,"
for example. Later published many poems and fifteen novels.

Morgan, John (1735–1789). M D, Edinburgh, 1767. Philadelphia
native who completed his education in Edinburgh and London. He became the first Professor of the Practice of Medicine at the University of Pennsylvania, where he helped
found the medical school. The improved plan for medical

education was based on Morgan's publication, *A Discourse Upon the Institution of Medical Schools in America* (Philadelphia, 1765).

Müller, Friedrich von (1858–1941). M D, Würzburg, LL D, McGill. Müller was inspired in physiological studies of clinical disorders by Carl von Voit in Munich and Carl Gerhardt at Würzburg. From Marburg, Müller reported the increase of metabolism in exophthalmic goiter in 1893. He returned to Munich in 1902 as Director of the 2nd Medical Clinic, where he established a world-famous center for clinical research. Dr. Karl Stauvli was one of his colleagues interested in research in clinical pathology.

Murphy, Daniel D. (1862–1931). Lawyer in Elkader, Iowa. L L D, Grinnell, Iowa, 1919. Member Iowa State Board of Education from its origin in 1909–25, and President of the Board, 1924–25.

Murphy, John B. (1857–1916). M D, Rush, 1879. LL D, Illinois, 1905. He trained in Chicago and Europe until 1887 when he became lecturer in surgery at Rush; professor of clinical surgery, College of Physicians and Surgeons, Chicago, 1894–1901; Professor of Surgery, Northwestern University, 1901–04, 1909–16, and at Rush, 1905–08. He was Chief Surgeon at Mercy Hospital, 1895–1916, and consultant at other hospitals in Chicago. His publications concerned the use of the "Murphy" button in anastomoses of the intestine, 1892; end-to-end suture of severed arteries and veins, 1897; surgery of the spinal cord, 1907, and arthroplasty and other surgical techniques for the skeletal system, 1912. He was president of the American Medical Association, 1910, and an honoree or member of other professional societies in America and abroad.

Neusser, Edmond von (1852–1912). Trained at Krakow and Vienna in internal medicine, he eventually was Professor and Director of the Second Medical Clinic, Vienna.

Noorden, Carl H. von (1858–1944). Professor of Medicine at Frankfurt until 1906 when he became Professor at Vienna. Studied disorders of the kidney, 1885, and also of metabolism. In 1910, he introduced a dietary treatment for diabetes.

Oertel, Horst (1873–1956). M D, Yale, 1894. Trained in Berlin and Leipzig, and worked in New York from 1907–14. Associate Professor, 1914–1920, and Professor of Pathology at McGill University, 1920–1939.

Olmsted, Ingersoll (1864–1936). M B, Toronto, 1887. Interned at German Hospital, Philadelphia, 1887–88. Fellow of American College of Surgeons and Royal College of Surgeons of Canada. Practiced at the General Hospital, Hamilton, Ontario.

Osborne, Marian G. (Mrs. H.C.) (1871–1931). Daughter of Osler's cousin, Marian Francis, and granddaughter of his uncle Edward Osler.

Osler, Sir Edmund Boyd (1845–1924). Brother of William Osler. Prominent Canadian financier. Interested in archeology, and a generous contributor to the Royal Ontario Museum. He also helped finance William Osler's early trips to Europe, and his later purchases of rare books.

Osler, Mrs. Featherstone Lake (née Ellen Free Pickton) (1806–1907). William Osler's mother. After her husband (1805–1895) retired and died in Toronto, she remained there with some of her family. Her 100th anniversary was celebrated as a near national occasion and the William Oslers were at her Toronto home with a large number of the extended family.

Packard, Francis R. (1870–1950). M D, Pennsylvania, 1892. Residency at Pennsylvania Hospital to 1895. A student and admirer of Osler. Professor at Philadelphia Polyclinic for

Graduates, 1901–1913. Served in World War I in France, 1917–1918. President of Medical Library Association, 1913. Edited *American Journal of the Medical Sciences,* 1901–06, and *Annals of Medical History,* 1919–42 (except for three years). Wrote *History of Medicine in the United States,* (1901–1931).

Parkin, Raleigh (c. 1895–   ). A youthful friend of Revere in Oxford, and the son of the secretary of the Rhodes Scholarship Trust, Sir George Parkin.

Parkinson, Sir John (1885–1976). M D, London, 1910. F.R.C.P., London. Chief Assistant to James Mackenzie, London Hospital, 1913–15. He was attached to the British Army Military Hospital at Hampstead in 1916, and in charge of the Army Heart Center, Rouen, France, 1917–1919. He was subsequently physician to the Cardiac Department, London Hospital, and the National Heart Hospital. He received many professional honors, and was knighted in 1948. Author of "Cardiac Disabilities of Soldiers in Active Service" (*Lancet* ii, 1916), and later articles on angina pectoris and other heart disorders.

Payne, Joseph Frank (1840–1910). M B, 1867; M D, Oxford. F.R.C.P., London. After training at St. George's Hospital and in Europe, he became Assistant Physician, 1873, and full Physician, 1887, at St. Thomas' Hospital. In addition to skill and publications in pathology, medicine and dermatology, he rose to prominence as a medical historian and book collector. He was Harveian Librarian of the Royal College of Physicians of London. His notable publications were on Anglo-Saxon and Anglo-Norman medicine. Their similar interests led to a close friendship with Osler.

Penfield, Wilder G. (1891–1976) B A, Oxford, 1916; M D, Johns Hopkins, 1918; Ph D, Oxford, 1935; Honorary D.Sc., Princeton, and many other honorary degrees and awards, including the Rhodes Scholarship. Engaged in research and neurosurgery at Columbia University and Presbyterian

Hospital, New York, 1921–28. Neurosurgeon to Royal Victoria and Montreal General Hospital, 1928–60; Director, Montreal Neurological Institute, 1934–60, and Professor, Neurology and Neurosurgery, McGill. Noted for physiologic and pathologic research by mapping areas of cerebral cortex. Numerous medical publications including *The Cerebral Cortex of Man* (1950), *Epilepsy and the Functional Anatomy of the Human Brain* (1954); also general literature. Penfield suffered an injury during a submarine attack in 1916, convalesced at "The Open Arms", and afterwards was an ardent disciple of Osler.

Pepper, William (1843–1898). M D, Pennsylvania, 1866. He was, in succession, Professor of Pathology, of Clinical Medicine, and of Practice of Medicine, 1868–98, and also Provost of the University of Pennsylvania, 1881–94. He wrote important medical articles and edited the first large *System of Medicine* (1886) in America.

Perkins, Mr. and Mrs. Charles, Burlington, Iowa. Mary was a daughter of Mrs. Perkins, who was a third cousin of Grace R. Osler.

Perley, Sir George Halsey (1857–1938). A member of the Canadian government, 1911–17; Minister of Overseas Military Forces of Canada, 1916–17. He was appointed High Commissioner for Canada and resided in London, 1914–22.

Peterson, Sir William (1856–1921). Educated in classics at Edinburgh and Corpus Christi College, Oxford. M A, D. Phil. Sc., LL D. He was teaching at Edinburgh, when appointed Principal of McGill University in 1895; retired in 1919. He was knighted in 1916.

Phillips, Llewellyn P. (1872–1927). M B, Cambridge, 1895; M D, F.R.C.S., F.R.C.P., London, Professor of Medicine, Egyptian Government Medical School, and Senior Physician,

Kasr-el-Ainy Hospital, Cairo, 1901–25. Effective work in cholera epidemic, 1901. He reported experiences with sandfly fever and the typhoid and paratyphoid fevers in Egypt, 1910. Published *Amoebiasis and the Dysenteries* (London, 1915).

Phipps, Henry (1839–1930). LL D, Pennsylvania, 1913. Industrialist and philanthropist. Interested in the tuberculosis movement. Gave Phipps Institute to the University of Pennsylvania, and the Phipps Psychiatric Hospital to Johns Hopkins.

Pollard, Alfred William (1859–1944). B A, Oxford, 1879, 1881. Librarian, bibliographer, and English scholar. He began work in 1883 in the printed books department at the British Museum, and was the Keeper, 1919–1924. Honorary Secretary, Bibliographical Society, 1893–1934; Honorary Professor of Bibliography, London University, 1919–32. He wrote and edited books on Shakespeare's works, and on early English printed books. Pollard also wrote the preface, and V. Scholderer of the Museum staff provided the bibliographic information, for William Osler: *Incunabula Medica: A Study of the Earliest Printed Medical Books* (1923).

Ponfick, Emil (1844–1913). Pathologist, trained at Berlin by R. Virchow, and later a Professor of Pathology at Breslau.

Pratt, Jospeh H. (1872–1956). MD, Johns Hopkins, 1898. Trained in pathology at Harvard under F. B. Mallory and W. T. Councilman, 1898–1902, and was also influenced in clinical research by Prof. Ludolf Krehl in Leipzig. From 1902 he combined private practice with laboratory investigation. He was Physician-in-Chief, Boston Dispensary, 1927–31, the New England Center Hospital, 1931–38, and the J. H. Pratt Diagnostic Hospital, 1938–56.

Prentiss, Henry James (1867–1931). M D, Bellevue Hospital Medical College, 1898. Taught in anatomy department at Bellevue,

1898–1904. Professor and Head of the Department of Anatomy, State University of Iowa, 1904–1931. He prepared excellent dissections, and was a gifted and inspiring teacher throughout his career. His interest in the applicability of anatomy to the treatment of disease prompted him to offer post-graduate courses. These courses were widely attended, and stimulated his students and colleagues in other departments to investigative research.

Pritchett, Henry S. (1857–1939). Astronomer and Educator. Ph.D. Munich, 1894. LL D, Hamilton College, 1900 and others. Superintendent U.S. Coast and Geodetical Survey, 1897–1900. President, Massachusetts Institute for Technology, 1900–06. President, Carnegie Foundation for Advancement of Teaching, 1906–30.

Raymond, Fulgence (1844–1910). M D, Paris, 1876. Succeeded his teacher, Charcot, at Salpêtrière as Professor in 1894. Published many articles on neurology.

Reese, D. Meredith (c. 1865–1892). M D, Pennsylvania, 1889. A student of Osler at Pennsylvania, he was an Assistant Resident Physician, Johns Hopkins Hospital, 1889–91. He became ill with pulmonary consumption and died at Saranac Lake.

Remsen, Ira D. (1846–1927). M D, College of Physicians and Surgeons, N.Y., 1867; Ph.D., Goettingen, 1870; LL D, Columbia, 1893 and others. Professor of Chemistry, 1876–1913, and President, 1901–12, Johns Hopkins University. Founded *American Chemical Journal*, 1879. Wrote numerous articles and books on chemistry.

Revere, Margaret A. (1896–   ), of Canton and Boston, Massachusetts. Daughter of Grace Osler's brother, Joseph W. Revere (1849–1932). Joseph's other children were Susan (1894–1947), Paul (1898–1972) and Anna (1900–1983).

Revere, Susan T. (Mrs. John) (1826–1911). Duaghter of John Gore Torrey and Susan Tilden. Her maternal great-grandfather was Capt. John Linzee of the British Navy. Her husband was a grandson of Paul Revere, and she was the mother of Joseph Revere, Grace Osler, Susan Chapin and Edward Revere.

Robb, A. Gardner (1866–1940). M B, Belfast; DPH. Physician, Belfast City Fever Hospital and Belfast Union Fever Hospital. He reported to the British Medical Association meeting in 1907: "Some observations on the recent outbreak of Cerebrospinal Fever in Belfast", *British Medical Journal*, ii (August 3, and October 26, 1907), pp. 286, 1129–31; also the following year he wrote on the treatment of this condition by Flexner's antimeningitis serum in *British Medical Journal*, i (February 15, 1908), pp. 382–86.

Roddick, Sir Thomas G. (1846–1923). M D, McGill, 1868. Professor of Surgery and Dean of Medicine, McGill, 1901–08; President of British Medical Association, 1897. Successfully promoted the Act for Uniform Medical Registration throughout Canada in 1912.

Rogers, Edmund James A. (1852–1922). M D, McGill, 1881. F.A.C.S. He was at school in Weston with Osler in 1867, and lived in the same house, 1877–81. He moved soon to Denver, Colorado; elected to American Climatological Society, 1890, and later was Professor of Surgery, University of Colorado.

Rolleston, Sir Humphry D. (1862–1944). Qualified in 1885; M D, Cambridge; LL D. After Research work at Cambridge, he was assistant, later physician to St. George's Hospital, London, 1898–1919; Regius Professor of Physic, Cambridge, 1925–32; President, Royal Society of Medicine, 1918–20 and of Royal College of Physicians, 1922–26. Editor, *Quarterly Journal of Medicine*, 1907–32. Wrote *Diseases of the Liver, Gall Bladder and Bile Ducts, The Cambridge Medical*

School; The Endocrine Glands in Health and Disease, and other works.

Ross, Frank William (1875–1966). Quebec business man who owned a trout fishing camp at Tantari, north of Quebec City, and salmon fishing rights in the Gaspé district.

Ross, James (1848–1918). British civil engineer who emigrated to North America in 1870. He participated in building Canadian Pacific Railway, 1883–85, and later was prominent financier in Montreal and abroad. He was a governor of McGill University and President of the Royal Victoria Hospital, to which he contributed the funds for the private patient pavillion. Mr. Ross was formerly a patient of Osler's friend, Arthur Browne.

Rowan, Charles J. (1874–1948). M D, Rush, 1898. After training in Chicago, Asia, and for a year, in Vienna, he was on J.B. Murphy's surgical staff at Cook County Hospital until 1906. He was then appointed assistant professor at Rush and Presbyterian Hospital, Chicago. In 1914, he became Professor and Head of Surgery at the University of Iowa, a post he held for sixteen years. He moved to Los Angeles, because of crippling arthritis, but his teaching abilities merited his appointment as Professor of Surgery, University of Southern California, 1931–39. Rowan and Howard were warm friends throughout their careers.

Rush, Benjamin (1745–1813). M D, Edinburgh, 1778. Pennsylvanian who was Professor of Chemistry in 1769, and held other chairs in the developing University of Pennsylvania. He was an able clinical teacher, as well as physician at the Pennsylvania Hospital, 1783–1813. Rush was one of the signers of the Declaration of Independence, and active in social causes. He is best remembered for a new approach to the management of insanity, for treating yellow fever patients in 1793 by copious bleeding, and for his "heroic" treatments in general medical practice.

Russel, Colin K. (1877–1956). M D, McGill, 1901. Interned at Royal Victoria Hospital, Montreal; trained in neurology at Johns Hopkins Hospital, 1902; under von Monakow in Zurich and elsewhere in Europe, 1903–04; Queens Square Hospital (London), 1905–06. Served in Canadian Army Medical Corps, 1915–19 and 1939–42. Clinical Professor of Neurology, McGill, 1922–36: Associate Professor, 1937–45. President, American Neurological Association, 1935.

Russell, J.S. Risien (1863–1939). M D, Edinburgh, 1886. F.R.C.P. Trained in neurology at the National Hospital, Queens Square, and in Europe before his brilliant experimental work in Horsley's Laboratory at the University College Hospital, London. He then became a leading clinical teacher and practitioner of neurology in London. Russell, et al, published a classical article on "Subacute Combined Degeneration of the Spinal Cord" (1900).

Sands, A. Collis (c. 1890–1917). An Oxford student who frequently visited "The Open Arms", and became close friends of the Oslers and their guests. He was killed in France during February, 1917.

Sargent, John Singer (1856–1925). LLD, Yale, 1916. Artist. Born of American parents in Italy. Studied painting in Florence and Paris. Opened studio in Paris, 1879. Resided in London, 1884–1925. Royal Academician, 1897. Visited the United States to exhibit paintings and paint portraits, 1876–1903. Famous for his portraits of President Theodore Roosevelt, and the Four Professors of Johns Hopkins Medical School— Welch, Osler, Halsted and Kelly.

Schmorl, C. Georg (1861–1932). M D, Professor at the Pathological Institute, Friedrichstadter Krankenhaus, Dresden. Introduced method for staining bone-sections in 1914.

Schorstein, Gustave Isidore (1863–1906). M B, Oxford, 1889; M D, 1904; F.R.C.P. Trained at Christ Church, Oxford, and Lon-

don Hospital, at which he was promoted to full Physician in
1905. He also served as Physician to Hospital for Consumption, Brompton. He was a talented physician and energetic
organizer at both the Oxford Medical School and London
Hospital School.

Servetus, Michael (c. 1511–1553). Spanish priest and physician who
wrote a book on religion, *Restitutio Christianismi* (1553).
Charged with heresy, he and most copies of his book were
burned by Calvinists. The book incidentally includes a brief
description of the circulation of blood through the lungs,
though scant evidence is offered to support this speculation.

Shepherd, Francis J. (1851–1929). M D, McGill, 1874; LL D, Harvard, McGill and Queens. Demonstrator, 1875, and Professor of Anatomy, 1883, McGill; Attending Surgeon, Montreal
General Hospital, 1885. Later, Surgeon-in-Chief at this hospital, Professor of Surgery and Dean of McGill College of
Medicine, 1908–14.

Sherrington, Charles S. (1857–1952). LL D. Fellow and President
of the Royal Society. He studied at Cambridge and St.
Thomas's Hospital to qualify, 1885. After two years in German Laboratories, he was made Lecturer at St. Thomas in
1887, and Professor at the Brown Institution, 1881. His
neurological experiments began there, and continued
while Professor at Liverpool, 1895–1913. He held the Chair
of Physiology at Oxford thereafter until he retired in 1930.
He was awarded the Nobel Prize in 1932. Among his chief
books were *The Integrative Action of the Nervous System*
(1906), *The Brain and its Mechanism* (1927), and *Reflex Activity of the Spinal Cord* (1932).

Shippen, William, Jr. (1736–1808). M D, Edinburgh, 1761. A Philadelphian, he was co-founder of the medical school of the
University of Pennsylvania and first Professor of Anatomy
and Surgery, 1765. He was Surgeon-General of the American forces, 1777–80.

Silliman, Benjamin (1779–1864). B A, Yale, 1796. Trained at Philadelphia and Princeton. Professor of Chemistry and Natural
History, Yale College, 1802–1853. He was an influential
member of the Committee to start the Yale Medical School,
of which he was the first Professor of Chemistry, 1813. Silliman wrote many scientific and literary articles and books.
In 1818, he founded and edited *The American Journal of
Sciences and Arts*. He achieved his greatest fame as a public
lecturer on geology and chemistry in Boston, New York,
and New Orleans. The Silliman Foundation at Yale is in
memory of Benjamin Silliman's sister-in-law, Mrs. Hepsa
Ely Silliman.

Singer, Charles J. (1876–1960). Qualified from Oxford and St.
Mary's Hospital, 1903. After further training in London and
abroad, he practiced medicine. He married Dorothea
Waley Cohen in 1910. In 1914, Singer began his career in
history with his wife at the Radcliffe Camera, Oxford. Active medical service in World War I interfered, but did not
stop his publications. From 1920 he was lecturer, and from
1931–42, Chairman of History of Medicine, University College, London. He received many professional honors. His
important publications include *Greek Biology and Greek
Medicine* (1922), *A Short History of Medicine* (1928), *A Short
History of Scientific Ideas to 1900* (1959). Dorothea Singer
collaborated with her husband, and also made her own contributions to medical history.

Smith, Nicola M. ("Miss Nichols") (1879–1954). Her family emigrated from Aberdeenshire to Indiana in 1892. She was Revere's governess in Baltimore, and for a short time, in Oxford. When he started school, she stayed on to help Grace
Osler entertain their guests. William Osler usually called
her "Miss Nichols," but apparently referred to her as "Scottie" in his January 14, 1907 letter to Marjorie Howard. Although not previously trained in office work, she typed
much of Osler's professional correspondence and remained
in Oxford through 1910. She then worked as a medical secretary in Baltimore until she retired to her birthplace in Scotland.

Somerville, Sir William (1860–1932). B Sc, Edinburgh; D Sc, Oxford; Fellow of Royal Society of Edinburgh. Professor of Rural Economy, Oxford, from 1902–25. Published books on trees and agriculture. The Somervilles were friends and neighbors of the Oslers.

Spies, Tom D. (1902–1960). M D, Harvard, 1928. Trained at Western Reserve, Cleveland to 1935; assistant and associate Professor of Medicine, University of Cincinnati, 1935–47; then Professor and Chairman of Nutrition and Metabolism, Northwestern Medical School, Chicago, 1947–60, but also directed clinical nutrition work at Hillman Hospital Birmingham, Alabama, starting in 1936. He is famous for his role in applying nicotinic acid treatment to pellagra in the Southern states, and later for being the first to use thiamine and folic acid for anemic diseases, especially the endemic anemias of Puerto Rico and Cuba. He received numerous honors from professional societies and the governments of the United States and Cuba.

Steindler, Arthur (1878–1959). M D, Vienna, 1902. F.A.C.S. Professor of Orthopaedics, Drake Medical School, Des Moines in 1910, before teaching at the State University of Iowa, Iowa City in 1912. He was appointed Professor in 1915, and became the first chairman of the separate Orthopaedic Department from 1927–1949. Then he continued practice as Professor Emeritus. He was President of the American Orthopaedic Association, and honored for his professional achievements in the United States, England, and elsewhere in America and Europe. His abilities as a clinician, innovator and organizer were embellished by his success in training his pupils in orthopaedics.

Stillé, Alfred (1813–1900). M D, Pennsylvania, 1836; LL D, 1889. Pupil of W.W. Gerhard at Philadelphia Hospital (Blockley), 1835–36, and then spent two years in Paris. Professor of Practice, 1854–64, and Professor of Medicine at Pennsylvania, 1864–84. President of American Medical Association, 1867. Writings included *Cerebrospinal Meningitis* (1867),

Materia Medica and Therapeutics: National Dispensatory.
Osler quoted Stillé: "Only two things are essential; to live
uprightly and to be wisely industrious."

Stokes, William (1804–1878). M D, Edinburgh, 1825. He wrote on
the use of Laënnec's stethoscope in diagnosis in 1825. Returning to Dublin, he succeeded his father as the Regius
Professor in 1845. With Robert Graves and others, the Dublin School attained fame for innovative clinical practice and
teaching. In 1846, William Stokes elaborated on Robert
Adams' earlier account of heart block. He also published on
typhus fever, cholera, and diseases of the lungs, heart and
aorta.

Strathcona and Mount Royal, Baron (Donald A. Smith) (1820–1914).
Born in Forres, Scotland, he joined The Hudson's Bay Company in Canada in his youth and gradually rose from a clerk
to governor by 1889. He was one of the principal organizers
of the Canadian Pacific Railway, a conservative politician,
and a successful financier. From 1896, until his death, he was
the British High Commissioner for Canada. He was made
a Baron in 1897, and lived in Great Britain. With his cousin,
he built and endowed the Royal Victoria Hospital, Montreal. He later built the College for Women, and provided
large funds for the Strathcona Medical Building and other
needs at McGill University. In his later years, he "raised a
regiment of rough-riders" in the Boer war, often answered
the appeals of Osler for projects in education and medicine,
and gave generously to Aberdeen University. He became
the Chancellor of Aberdeen and McGill Universities.

Strong, Richard P. (1872–1948). M D, Tufts, 1897. Intern, Johns
Hopkins Hospital, 1897–98. Professor of Tropical Medicine,
Harvard University. While in U.S. Medical Corps, A.E.F.,
was chief author of *Trench Fever* (1918). Subsequently,
he returned to Harvard. He also became Colonel, M.D.,
Consultant to the Secretary of War, and Director of
Tropical Medicine, Army Medical School, Washington,
D.C.

Sydenham, Thomas (1624–1689). M B, Oxford, 1648. He served in Cromwell's cavalry during, and after, his undergraduate education. Completed training at Montpellier, 1661; M D, Cambridge, 1676. He practiced in London, and gained a wide reputation throughout Europe as "The English Hippocrates". His attentive observation of the clinical manifestations in individual patients led him to classical descriptions of such diseases as gout, measles, pneumonia and the prevailing intermittent fever. He noted that the latter fever responded to the Peruvian bark (i.e., quinine). Thus his writings set the stage for the 19th century concepts of specific diseases and treatments.

Tait, John (1878–1944). M D, Edinburgh, 1903; Fellow of Royal Society; Professor of Physiology, McGill, 1929–40. Honored in Britain and North America for his original research on the physiology of nerves, circulation, the inner ear and other systems.

Thayer, William S. (1864–1932). M D, Harvard, 1889. LL D, Edinburgh and others. Resident physician, 1891–98, and Associate in Medicine, Johns Hopkins Hospital, 1899–1905. Then pursued his practice, and served on the faculty of clinical medicine until distinguished World War I service from 1917–19. Professor and Head of Medicine, Johns Hopkins, 1919, until April 1921, when he resigned to resume practice and Clinical Professorship. Many military and professional honors and society memberships. President, American Medical Association, 1928. Author of *Lectures on Malarial Fevers* (1897), and other medical and educational topics.

Thomas, Henry M. (1861–1925). M D, Maryland, 1885. The son of a Trustee of Johns Hopkins University, Dr. James Carey Thomas, and a brother of Miss M. Carey Thomas. She was a leader in the Women's Fund Committee which raised the necessary money, with Mary Garrett's generosity, to open the Medical school in 1893. Henry Thomas joined the Johns Hopkins Hospital out-patient staff for neurology in 1889, and in 1896 was appointed Clinical Professor of Diseases of the Nervous System. He remained in charge of this division of the Department of Medicine until his death. He served as President of the American Neurological Society in 1910.

Tizzoni, Guido (1853–1932). M D. Professor of Pathology, Bologna, until 1928. Contributed especially to bacteriology and immunity, including the independent preparation of anti-tetanus serum. During 1908–1915, reported investigations on pellagra in support of its bacterial etiology.

Toulmin, Harry (1865–1929). M D, Pennsylvania, 1889. A student of Osler's in Philadelphia, and the first assistant resident physician at Johns Hopkins Hospital, 1889–90. He practiced medicine in Philadelphia until his death.

Trudeau, Edward, L. (1848–1915). M D, College of Physicians and Surgeons, New York, 1871. L L D, McGill and Pennsylvania. Two years after graduation, he suffered pulmonary tuberculosis, but he improved in the Adirondacks. In 1884, he founded the first fresh air sanatorium for pulmonary tuberculosis in the United States at Saranac Lake, New York. He wrote many articles on controlling this disease, and was the first president of the National Association for the Prevention of Tuberculosis in 1905.

Turner, Lieutenant General Sir Richard E.W. (1871–1961), VC, KCB, KCMG. Won Victoria Cross during the Boer War in South Africa in 1901. Promoted to Major General while serving in France, and assumed command of Canadian Forces in Britian in December, 1916. He was again promoted and served as Chief of the General Staff, Overseas Military Forces of Canada, from May 18, 1918 until November 22, 1919.

Tyson, James (1841–1919). M D, Pennsylvania, 1863. Professor of Pathology, 1876–89; Professor of Clinical Medicine, 1889–

99, and Professor of Medicine, University of Pennsylvania, 1899–1910. President of the Association of American Physicians, 1907–08. Writings included *The Cell Doctrine, Its History and Present State*, (1870), *The Practice of Medicine. A Textbook* . . . (1896).

Van Epps, Clarence E. (1875–1962). M D, Iowa, 1897, and Pennsylvania, 1898. He taught at Iowa University from 1900 to retirement as Assistant, Associate and Professor of Medicine, Professor of Therapeutics, and Professor of Neurology. Served in World War I. He was a member of the Central Society for Clinical Research, Association for Research in Nervous and Mental Disorders, and Central Neuropsychiatric Association.

Verdon, Francis. Trained at King's College Hospital; qualified 1888. Served as surgeon on British passenger ships until about 1912. Retired thereafter from medical practice in London.

Vesalius, Andreas (1514–1564). M D, Padua, 1537. Born in Brussels, he studied anatomy under Jacques Dubois (Sylvius) at Paris before he completed his training at Padua. With illustrations by Jan van Kalkar of Titian's school, Vesalius published the first accurate text on human anatomy, *De humani corporis fabrica libri septem* (Basel, 1542). Realdo Colombo (1516–1559), and Andreas Cesalpinus (1524–1603) were Italians who contributed to knowledge of the heart's action.

Villemin, Jean-Antoine (1827–1892). M D, Paris, 1853. Later military physician, then Medical Inspector of the Army. Wrote on tuberculosis "De tubercule au point de vue de son siége, de son évolution and de sa nature" (1862); its virulence, "Causes et nature de la tuberculose" (1866); and its specificity, "Études sur la tuberculose, prueves rationelles et expérimentelles de la spécificité et de son inoculabilité" (1868).

Virchow, Rudolf (1821–1902). M D, Berlin, 1843. As founder of the
doctrine of cellular pathology, 1858, epitomized by "omnis
cellula e cellula", he made such important and numerous
contributions to pathology to be a leading figure in world-
wide medicine. He also contributed greatly to hygiene,
epidemiology, social reform, anthropology and archeology.
In addition to his own publications he insituted the *Archiv
für pathologische Anatomie* (1847–   ), which now bears
his name. Osler carefully recorded Virchow's autopsies in
Berlin during the autumn of 1873, visited him again in 1884,
and always admired his work.

Wagstaffe, William W. (1886–1928). M B, Oxford, 1911. F.R.C.S. At
New College, Oxford, he studied the works of Vesalius and
other early anatomists with Osler and gained a first class
degree in Natural Science, 1908. Trained in surgery at St.
Thomas Hospital, he had extensive surgical experience in
World War I. Practiced in Oxford from 1921, andpromoted
to Surgeon at Radcliffe Infirmary, 1927. He was an early
member of the Osler Club in London, and left valuable
books to its library.

Walton, Izaak (1593–1683). English author of a famous book on
fishing and outdoor life, *The Compleat Angler, or the Con-
templative Man's Recreation,* 1653.

Warthin, Alfred Scott (1866–1931) M D, Michigan, 1891 and Ph D,
1893. Trained in medicine and pathology. Promoted to Director and Professor of Pathology, University of Michigan
Medical School, 1903–31. President of several pathological
societies and editor of journals, and a founder of the *Bulletin of International Association of Medical Museums.* He
described traumatic lipemia and fatty embolism (1913), and
methods for demonstrating spirochaetes in tissues (1920–21).

Warthin, Thomas A. (1909–   ). M D, Harvard, 1934. Internist.
Presently at Veterans' Administration Hospital, 810 Nepon-
set Street, Norwood, Massachusetts, 02062.

Welch, William H. (1850–1934). M D, College of Physicians and Surgeons, New York, 1875. LL D of many universities. Imbued with German methods of medical science, he taught successfully in New York, 1876–84. Though appointed professor of Pathology at Johns Hopkins he studied bacteriology in Germany for a year until 1885. He was Professor of Pathology for thirty-three years, Director of the School of Hygiene and Public Health, 1920–29, and Professor of the History of Medicine, 1929–34, at Johns Hopkins. Welch's leadership in American medical science is evident by his influential advice to the Rockefeller Medical Institutions. He was also president of the Association of American Physicians, 1902, American Association of Pathologists and Bacteriologists, 1906, American Medical Association, 1911, American Social Hygiene Association, 1916–19, the American Association of the History of Medicine, 1927, and many others.

Wenckebach, Karl Friedrich (1864–1940). M D, Utrecht, 1888. Professor of Internal Medicine, Gröningen, 1900–11, and Strasburg, 1911–14. Then he was an associate with von Noorden at University of Vienna Medical Clinic, and concluded his career as a Professor at Vienna. He wrote on many subjects, but is famous for articles on cardiac arrhythmias (1903–1914), and on the origin of pain in coronary sclerosis (1928).

White, James William (1850–1916). M D, University of Pennsylvania, 1871; LL D, Aberdeen, 1900. Professor of Surgery, University of Pennsylvania and Surgeon at University Hospital until 1910, then Emeritus. Author of many articles and co-author with W.W. Keen of *American Textbook of Surgery* (1896).

Whitehead, Richard H. (1865–1916). M D, Virginia, 1887. Professor of Anatomy and Dean of Medicine, North Carolina, 1891–1905. Professor of Anatomy and Dean of Medicine, Virginia, Charlottesville, 1905–16. Member of AMA conferences on medical education. Author of *Anatomy of the Brain*.

Whitnall, Samuel Ernest (1876–1950). M B, Oxford, 1902; M A, M
D, and Demonstrator at Oxford. Professor of Anatomy,
McGill, 1919–1935; Professor of Anatomy, Bristol University,
1935–1941; Fellow of Royal Society (Canada). Several scientific publications, and *The Study of Anatomy* (1922; ed. 4,
1939).

Williams, J. Whitridge (1886–1931). M D, Maryland, 1888. LL D. He
trained in Germany and Austria for a year. Became Associate in Gynecology, Johns Hopkins Hospital, 1890, and in
1895 his title was changed to indicate his responsibility for
teaching obstetrics. Professor of Obstetrics from 1899–1931;
Dean of Medicine from 1911–1923, and chairman of the full-
time obstetrics department from 1919–1931. He was President of American Gynecological Society, 1913–14, and of the
American College of Surgeons, 1914–16. He described papil-
lary cystomata of the ovary (1891), deciduoma malignum
(1895), and wrote *Textbook of Obstetrics* (1913, 6th ed., 1930).

Wilson, James C. (1847–1934). M D, Jefferson, 1869. Professor of the
Practice of Medicine and Clinical Medicine, Jefferson Medical College, President of the Associatiion of American
Physicians, 1902. He wrote *A Handbook of Medical Diagnosis* (1909), and edited *American Textbook of Applied Therapeutics.*

Wood, Horatio C. (1841–1920). M D, Pennsylvania, 1862. L L D,
LaFayette, Yale and Pennsylvania. At various times he was
Professor of botany, nervous disorders and materia medica,
University of Pennsylvania, 1866–1907. Among his published experiments on animals and man was one on the
action of atropine to block the fall of blood pressure in
shock. He edited the *United States Dispensatory* (1883–
1907).

Wright, Henry P. (1851–1899). M D, McGill, 1871. Shared rooms
with Osler in Montreal from 1870–71. After a year's study in
London and elsewhere, he established his practice in Ot-

tawa in 1872. He was President of the Canadian Medical Association in 1889, and of the Ottawa Medical Society in 1896. He died in 1899 from acute "angina pectoris" (probably myocardial infarction).

Wright, Mrs. Henry P. (Marion Grahame, 1861–1945). A daughter of Scottish settlers near modern Toronto, she married Dr. Wright of Ottawa in 1887. After her husband's sudden death, the Oslers continued their friendship with her and her seven children in Canada, and later in England. During World War I, Mrs. Wright rented a house near the Oslers in Oxford from September 1915, but she moved to London in 1918.

Wright, Henry P.G. (1888–1952). M D, McGill, 1913. Eldest son of H.P. Wright, M.D. of Ottawa. Married Nora Blake. A member of the Canadian Army Medical Corps 1914–18, including service in France, and Special Hospitals in England studying nerve shock after September, 1916. He saw Osler frequently during World War I, and was a principal founder of the Osler Reporting Society in Montreal in 1920. From 1919–1941, he practiced pediatrics at the Children's Memorial and Royal Victoria Hospitals. After further military duty in Montreal during World War II, he resumed practice in rheumatology, and was a leading advocate of, and participant in, occupational therapy schools in Canada.

Wright, Jean (1894–   ). Third daughter of H.P. Wright, Jean accompanied her mother and sisters to Oxford in September, 1915, and worked as a volunteer nurse in Canadian Army Hospitals. She married Major Allen P.O. Meredith at Oxford on Jan. 4, 1919.

Wright, Miss Marion Gertrude (1896–   ). Fourth daughter of H.P. Wright. She accompanied her mother to Oxford in 1915, and soon worked as a volunteer nurse in Army hospitals. Later she worked on English farms. She was the same age and a friend of Revere Osler.

Wright, Palmer (1891–1952). Second son of H.P. Wright, he was an officer with the Canadian artillery in France during World War I.

Wright, Mrs. Palmer (1891–1980). Hilda was a daughter of Sir Percy Sherwood of Ottawa. She married during June 1915 while her husband was in the Canadian army, and went to Oxford with Mrs. H.P. Wright in September, 1915.

Wright, Phoebe (1890–1972). Eldest daughter of Dr. and Mrs. H.P. Wright. She preceded her mother to England in 1915, and was a volunteer nurse with Canadian Army Hospitals in Britain and France from 1915 through 1918. She married Captain Reginald Fitz, U.S. A.M.C. at Oxford on June 29, 1918.

Wright, Lieutenant William R. (1898–1917). Youngest son of H.P. Wright, M.D. After brief service in England, he was posted to the Canadian Infantry in France on April 26, 1917, and killed on May 13.

Yates, Lieutenant Colonel Henry B. (1865–1916). M D, McGill, 1893. Assistant in bacteriology at Royal Victoria Hospital and McGill. Affiliated with Army Medical Service in Canada from 1894 to 1915. Joined No. 3 Canadian General Hospital in April, 1915 as Lieutenant Colonel.

Young, Hugh H. (1870–1945). M D, Virginia, 1894. After two years of pathology and internship, he joined Johns Hopkins Hospital as assistant resident surgeon in 1896, and was placed in charge of genitourinary diseases in the dispensary in 1897. In 1908 he was appointed associate in surgery, a post he held until 1914. The next year he became Clinical Professor of Urology and Director of the Brady Urological Institute at Johns Hopkins where he remained until his retirement in 1942. He served as Chief of Urology with the U.S. Army in France from 1917. Though best known as the organizer of his specialty, and the teacher of numerous academic and practicing urologists, he was extremely active in writing. He was President of the American Urological Association. Among his many urological publications were noteworthy reports on surgical management of hermaphroditism.

Appendices

Robert Palmer Howard, M.D. (1823–1889)—Bibliography

"A Clinical Lecture on the Diagnosis of Cardiac Disease". *Canada Medical Journal and Monthly Record of Medical and Surgical Science* 1 (1852): pp. 265–274; "A Few Observations on Dr. Howard's Lecture", by Medicus. *Ibid.:* pp. 343–46; "Review of a Few Observations on Dr. Howard's Lecture by Medicus", by R.P.H. *Ibid.:* pp. 407–09.

"Severe Constrictive Disease of the Mitral Valve and Orifice, Without a Direct but With an Indirect Mitral Murmur, Nonpersistent, and Probably of Dynamic Origin, with Remarks." *The Medical Chronicle* 1 (1853): pp. 5–7; *ibid.:* pp. 38–41.

"Removal of an Encysted Tumor, Which Resembled a Hernia in Several Particulars, with Remarks". *The Medical Chronicle* 1 (1854): pp. 222–25.

"Lecture on a Case of Aneurism of Arch of Aorta and Diseased Heart, delivered in March 1853". *The Medical Chronicle* 2 (1855): pp. 41–46; "Sequel to Lecture . . . , with Observations." *Ibid.:* pp. 87–92.

"On Gangrene of the Lungs". *The Medical Chronicle* 5 (1857): pp. 49–59.

"Clinical Lecture on Inflammation and Perforation of the Appendix Vermiformis." *The Medical Chronicle* 5 (1858): pp. 527–38.

"Two Examples of Myeloid Tumor: with General Observations upon that Form of Growth, read before the Medical Students' Society of McGill College." *The Medical Chronicle* 6 (1859): pp. 433–42; *ibid.:* pp. 485–95.

"Case of True Leprosy, with Brief Remarks." *Canada Medical Journal* 5 (1868): pp. 151–56.

"Valedictory Address to the Graduates in Medicine, delivered on May 4, 1869." *Canada Medical Journal* 5 (1869): pp. 529–35.

"The First Epidemic of Cerebro-Spinal Fever in Montreal". *Canada Medical And Surgical Journal* 1 (1872): pp. 97–106.

180   *Appendices*

"President's Address. Read Before the Medico-Chirurgical Society, Oct. 19, 1872". *Canada Medical And Surgical Journal* 1 (1872): pp. 224–28.

"Some Observations Upon Scarlatinal Pleurisy and Upon Thoracentesis in That Affection. Read before the Canadian Medical Association in September 1872." *Canada Medical and Surgical Journal* 1 (1872): pp. 241–46.

"Cases of Fibrous Polypi and Fibrous Tumours of the Uterus. Read before the Medico-Chirurgical Society on 13th June, 1873." *Canada Medical and Surgical Journal* 2 (1873): pp. 1–12.

"Introductory Lecture Delivered at the Opening of the Forty-First Session of the Medical Faculty of McGill University." *Canada Medical and Surgical Journal* 2 (1873): pp. 193–212.

"Objections to Some of the Recent Views Upon the Pathology of Tubercle and Pulmonary Consumption, being the Address in Medicine read before the Canadian Medical Association." *Canada Medical and Surgical Journal* 3 (1874): pp. 97–107.

"Some Observations on the Preceding Case of Cerebro-Spinal Meningeal Haemorrhage." *Canada Medical and Surgical Journal* 3 (1875): pp. 487–92.

"Report from Canada," *Annual Report on the Diseases of the Chest* . . . , ed. H. Dobell, 1874–75, Vol. I. London, 1875, pp. 233–42.

"Cases of Pernicious Progressive Anaemia, with Some Observations Upon the Ante- and Post-Mortem Conditions Observed in that Affection", in *Transactions of the International Medical Congress of Philadelphia.* Edited for the Congress by John Ashhurst, Jr., A.M., M.D. Philadelphia, 1877, pp. 443–51.

"Two Cases of Stenosis of the Tricuspid Orifice with Observations." *Transactions of the Canada Medical Association* (Tenth Annual Meeting), 1 (1877): pp. 110–18.

"A Clinical Lecture Upon a Case of Contraction of the Right Side of the Chest and Great Enlargement of the Superior Half of the Abdomen". *Canada Medical and Surgical Journal* 7 (1879): pp. 241–54.

"Inaugural Address at the Medico-Chirugical Society of Montreal". *Canada Medical and Surgical Journal* 8 (1879): pp. 193–99.

"Cases of Leucocythemia." *Montreal General Hospital Reports* 1 (1880): pp. 1–44.

"A Case of Fibroid Disease of the Heart with Observations upon the General Pathology of Fibrosis." *Canada Medical and Surgical Journal* 8 (1880): pp. 529–44.

"The President's Address. Delivered before the Canada Medical Association at its 13th Annual Meeting at Ottawa". *Canada Medical and Surgical Journal* 9 (1880): pp. 65–82.

"Valedictory Address to the Graduating Class." *Canada Medical and Surgical Journal* 9 (1881): pp. 513–21.

"Some Observations upon the International Congress". *Canada Medical and Surgical Journal* 10 (1881): pp. 144–54.

"The Introductory Address of the Fiftieth Session of the Medical Faculty of McGill University. A Sketch of the History of the Faculty and of the Life of the Late Dean, G. W. Campbell, A.M., M.D., LL. D," in *Medical Faculty, McGill College. Semi-Centennial Celebration.* Montreal, 1882, pp. 1–24.

"On some of the Varieties of Dyspnoea Met With in Bright's Disease, read before the Canada Medical Association, Montreal, 1884." *Canada Medical and Surgical Journal* 13 (1884): pp. 193–200.

"Rheumatism", in *A System of Practical Medicine by American Authors*, edited by W. Pepper and L. Starr, vol. II. Philadelphia, Lea Brothers & Co., 1885, pp. 19–107.

"On Hepatic Cirrhosis in Children". *Transactions of the Association of American Physicians* 2 (1887): pp. 1–36; also, a shorter version, *American Journal of Medical Sciences* 94 (1887): pp. 350–63.

"Case of Bilateral Ophthalmoplegia Externa and Interna Associated with Tabes Dorsalis, Bulbar Paralysis, and Loss of Vision and Hearing. With some observations upon the Pathogeny and Etiology of Bilateral Ophthalmoplegia Externa." *American Journal of the Medical Sciences* 97 (1889): pp. 238–47.

Notes on Practice of Medicine [revised transcript of R.P. Howard's Lectures, with few additions by Dr. Geo. Ross]. Montreal, 1891.

Campbell P. Howard, M.D.—Bibliography

Howard, C.P. "A Case of Quartan Malaria." *Montreal Medical Journal* 31 (March, 1902): pp. 179–81.

Howard, C.P. "Pneumococcic Arthritis: Report of Three Cases." *Johns Hopkins Hospital Bulletin* 14 (November, 1903): pp. 303–06.

Howard, C.P. "The Incidence of Gastric Ulcer in America." *Medical News* 85 (October 8, 1904): pp. 673–75.

Howard, C.P. "A Study of Ulcer of the Stomach and Duodenum: Based Upon a Series of Eighty-Two Cases." *American Journal of the Medical Sciences* 128 (December, 1904): pp. 939–66.

Howard, C.P. "Gastric Ulcer: Clinical Varieties and Symptoms." *Johns Hopkins Hospital Bulletin* 16 (March, 1905): p. 116.

Howard, C.P. "Symptomatology and Diagnosis of Gastric Ulcer." *Proceedings of the Philadelphia County Medical Society* 26 (1905): pp. 125–31.

Howard, C.P. "Gastric Tetany." *Johns Hopkins Hospital Bulletin* 16 (April, 1905): p. 148.

Howard, C.P. "Tetany: A report of Nine Cases." *American Journal of the Medical Sciences* 131 (1906): pp. 301–29.

Howard, C.P. "Myxedema: A Study." *Journal of the American Medical Association* 48 (April 13, April 20, April 27, 1907): pp. 1226–30; 1325–33; 1403–08.

182   *Appendices*

Howard, C.P. "Serum Sickness and Serum Death: A Compilation of Some Recent Literature." *Montreal Medical Journal* 36 (September, 1907): pp. 610–15

Howard, C.P. "The Relation of the Eosinophilic Cells of the Blood, Peritoneum and Tissues to Various Toxins." *Journal of Medical Research* 17 (December, 1907): pp. 237–69.

Howard, C.P. "Mikulicz's Disease and Allied Conditions." *International Clinics* 1 (1909): pp. 31–64.

Howard, C.P. "The Chemistry of the Urine in Diabetes Mellitus." *American Journal of the Medical Sciences* 137 (May, 1909): pp. 715–24.

Howard, C.P. "Pneumococcic Arthritis". *Johns Hopkins Hospital Reports* 15 (1910): pp. 229–45.

Howard, C.P. "The First Annual Report of the St. George's Tuberculosis Class." Montreal: privately printed, 1910.

Howard, C.P. "Living Cases (Microcephalic Idiocy and True Amaurotic Idiocy)." *Montreal Medical Journal* 39 (June, 1910): pp. 428–32.

Duval, C.W. and Howard, C.P. "Chronic Aleucemic Enlargement of the Lymphatic Glands." *Archives of Internal Medicine* 5 (January, 1910): pp. 6–21.

Howard, C. P. "Some Common Types of Coma." *Iowa Medical Journal* 17 (January 15, 1911): pp. 343–56.

Howard, C.P. "Some Unusual Complications of Typhoid Fever." *Iowa Medical Journal* 18 (July 15, 1911): pp. 1–17.

Howard, C.P. "Etiology and Pathogenesis of Anemia." *Journal of the Iowa State Medical Society* 1 (October, 1911): pp. 169–80.

Howard, C.P. "The Treatment of Acute Lobar Pneumonia." *Journal of the Iowa State Medical Society* 1 (November, 1911): pp. 262–65.

Howard, C.P. and Wolbach, S.B. "Congenital Obliteration of the Bile Ducts." *Archives of Internal Medicine* 8 (November, 1911): pp. 557–73.

Baumann, L. and Howard, C.P. "Metabolism of Scurvy in an Adult." *Transactions of the Association of American Physicians* 27 (1912): pp. 514–23; also, *Archives of Internal Medicine* 9 (June, 1912): pp. 665–79.

Howard, C.P. "Some Points in the Etiology and Recognition of Aortic Insufficiency." *Journal of the Iowa State Medical Society* 2 (October, 1912): pp. 247–54.

Howard, C.P. "Spondylitis Deformans." *Iowa Medical Journal* 19 (May 15, 1913): pp. 577–86.

Howard, C.P. "Differential Diagnosis of Diseases of the Upper Abdominal Quadrants." *Journal of the Iowa State Medical Society* 2 (June 1, 1913): pp. 864–71.

Howard, C.P. "The Etiology and Pathogenesis of Bronchiectasis." *Transactions of the Association of American Physicians* 28 (1913): pp. 758–80; also, *American Journal of Medical Sciences* 147 (March, 1914): pp. 313–32.

Howard, C.P. "The Medical Aspects of Sarcoma." *Journal of the Iowa State Medical Society* 4 (July, 1914): pp. 12–22; also, *Iowa Medical Journal* 20 (1914): pp. 467–72.

Howard, C.P. "Diagnosis of Tumors of the Mediastinum." *Medical Herald* [Kansas City, Missouri] 33 (November, 1914): pp. 417–22.

Howard, C.P. "The Diagnosis of Mediastinitis." *Johns Hopkins Hospital Bulletin* 26 (May, 1915): pp. 140–44; annotation, *Lancet* ii (August 14, 1915): pp. 350–51.

Howard, C.P. "The Physical Signs and Symptoms of Wounds of the Chest." *Transactions of the Association of American Physicians* 31 (1916): pp. 65–78; also, with modified title, *American Journal of the Medical Sciences* 152 (November, 1916): pp. 650–60.

Howard, C.P. and Royce, C.E. "Progressive Lenticular Degeneration Associated with Cirrhosis of the Liver (Wilson's Disease)." *Transactions of the Association of American Physicians* 32 (1917): pp. 460–78; also, *Archives of Internal Medicine* 24 (November, 1919): pp. 497–508.

Baumann, L. and Howard, C.P. "The Mineral Metabolism of Experimental Scurvy of the Guinea-pig." *American Journal of the Medical Sciences* 153 (May, 1917): pp. 650–65.

Howard, C.P. and Ingvaldsen, T. "The Mineral Metabolism of Experimental Scurvy of the Monkey." *Johns Hopkins Hospital Bulletin* 28 (July, 1917): pp. 222–25.

Howard, C. P. and Stevens, F.A. "The Iron Metabolism of Hemochromatosis." *Archives of Internal Medicine* 20 (December 1917): pp. 896–912.

Howard, C.P. "Some of the Medical Lessons of the Present War." *Journal of the Iowa State Medical Society* 8 (October, 1918): pp. 351–55.

Hansmann, G. H. and Howard, C.P. "Urobilin and Urobilinogen of Stool and Urine in Pernicious Anemia: Their Value in Diagnosis and Prognosis." *Journal of the American Medical Association* 73 (October 25, 1919): pp. 1262–64.

Howard, C.P. "Functional Diagnosis of Polyglandular Disease in Acromegaly and Other Disturbances of the Hypohysis." *Transactions of the Association of American Physicians* 34 (1919): pp. 271–83; also, *American Journal of Medical Sciences* 158 (December, 1919): pp. 830–39.

Howard, C.P. "The Clinical Aspects of the Pneumonia of Influenza". *Contributions to Medical and Biological Research, Dedicated to Sir William Osler . . . in Honour of his 70th Birthday . . .* , vol. 1, pp. 575–81. New York: P.B. Hoeber, 1919.

Howard, C.P. "Diseases of the Salivary Glands". In *Nelson Loose-Leaf Medicine,* vol. 5, pp. 21–33. New York: Thomas Nelson & Sons, 1920.

Howard, C. P. "Obesity". In *The Oxford Medicine,* vol. 4, edited by H. A. Christian and J. MacKenzie, pp. 195–213. New York: Oxford University Press, 1921.

Howard, C.P. "Hemochromatosis". *Ibid.*, pp. 215–22.

Howard, C.P. "Ochronosis". *Ibid.*, pp. 223–28.

Howard, C.P. "Rickets". *Ibid.*, pp. 229–52.

Howard, C.P. "Scurvey". *Ibid.*, pp. 253–72.

Gibson, R.B. and Howard, C.P. "A Case of Alkaptonuria with a Study of its Metabolism." *Transactions of the Association of American Physicians* 36 (1921): pp. 258–65; *Archives of Internal Medicine* 28 (November, 1921): pp. 632–37.

Howard, C. P. "Treatment of Pneumonia with Special Reference to the Use of Serum." *Canadian Medical Association Journal* 11 (October, 1921): pp. 709–13.

Howard, C.P. "Clinical Syndromes Due to Thyroid Disease". In *Endocrinology and Metabolism*, vol. 1, edited by L.F. Barker, pp. 229–377. New York: D. Appleton and Co., 1922.

Howard, C. P. "The Passing of the Medical Practitioner." *Journal of the Iowa State Medical Society* 12 (January, 1922): pp. 1–6.

Howard, C.P. "Some Phases of Dysthyroidism". *Canadian Medical Association Journal* 12 (September, 1922): pp. 606–09.

Howard, C. P. "The Relation of the State University Hospital to the Medical Profession". *Journal of the American Medical Association* 80 (May 12, 1923): pp. 1401–02.

Gibson, R.B. and Howard, C. P. "The Chemistry of Pseudochylous Ascites and Other Types of Exudates". *American Journal of the Medical Sciences* 166 (July, 1923): pp. 80–89.

Gibson, R. B. and Howard, C. P. "Metabolic Studies in Pernicious Anemia". *Archives of Internal Medicine* 32 (July, 1923): pp. 1–16.

Howard, C. P. "Pulmonary Syphilis". *The American Journal of Syphilis* 8 (January, 1924): pp. 1–33.

Howard, C.P. "Diseases of the Lymphatic Glands". In *Billings-Forchheimer Therapeusis of Internal Disease*, 4th ed., rev., edited by George Blumer, pp. 922–36. New York: D. Appleton and Company, 1924.

Howard, C.P. "Periarteritis Nodosa: A Review of Our Knowledge". *Canadian Medical Association Journal* 15 (May, 1925): pp. 473–75.

Howard, C.P. "The Sphere of the Dietitian". *Journal of the American Dietetic Association* 2 (June, 1926): pp. 1–5.

Howard, C.P. and Rabinowitch, I.M. "Guanidine Excretion in Relation to Hypertension". *Journal of Clinical Investigation* 2 (August, 1926): pp. 587–92.

Howard, C.P. "Recollections of Sir William Osler's Visit to No. 3 Canadian General Hospital (McGill)". Sir William Osler Memorial Number, Appreciations and Reminiscences, Second Impression. *Bulletin of the International Association of Medical Museums* 9 (1926): pp. 419–20.

Osler, W., revised by Howard, C.P. "Diseases of the Arteries". In *Modern Medicine: Its Theory and Practice*, edited by W. Osler and re-edited by T. McCrae and E.H. Funk, vol. 4, pp. 813–39. Philadelphia: Lea & Febiger, 1927.

Osler, W., revised by Howard, C.P. "Aneurism". *Ibid.*, pp. 840–92.

Howard, C.P. "The Incidence and Clinical Diagnosis of Acute Yellow Atrophy of the Liver". *Transactions of the Association of American Physicians* 42 (1927): pp. 140–65; also, *Canadian Medical Association Journal* 17 (September, 1927): pp. 996–1005.

Howard, C.P. and Mills, E.S. "Acute Articular Rheumatism and Other Members of the Rheumatic Cycle". *Canadian Medical Association Journal* 19 (October, 1928): pp. 403–11.

Howard, C.P. "Aortic Insufficiency Due to Rupture by Strain of A Normal Aortic Valve." *Canadian Medical Association Journal* 19 (July, 1928): pp. 12–24.

Howard, C.P. "The President's Address". *Transactions of the Association of American Physicians* 44 (1929): pp. 1–6.

Howard, C.P. and Mills, E.S. "Obesity". In *The Oxford Medicine*, vol. 4, edited by H. A. Christian, pp. 195–214 (1). New York: Oxford University Press, 1929.

Howard, C.P. and Mills, E.S. "Haemochromatosis". *Ibid.*, pp. 215–22.

Howard, C. P. and Mills, E.S. "Ochronosis". *Ibid.*, pp. 223–28.

Howard, C.P. and Mills, E.S. "Rickets". *Ibid.*, pp. 229–52 (2).

Howard, C.P. and Mills, E.S. "Scurvy". *Ibid.*, pp. 253–71.

Howard, C.P. *The Diagnosis and Treatment of Pneumonia.* Oxford Monographs on Diagnosis and Treatment, vol. 10, edited by H. A. Christian. New York: Oxford University Press, 1931.

Howard, C.P. "A Medical Clinic". *Journal of the Iowa State Medical Society* 21 (August, 1931): pp. 425–38.

Howard, C.P. and Fullerton, C.W. "A Study of Cancer of the Stomach". *Canadian Medical Association Journal* 27 (September, 1932): pp. 227–36.

Howard, C.P. and Fullerton, C.W. "The Treatment of Lobar Pneumonia". *Canadian Medical Association Journal* 27 (October, 1932): pp. 367–71.

Howard, C. P. and Mills, E.S. "A Study of So-Called Splenic Anemia and Banti's Syndrome". *Transactions of the Association of American Physicians* 47 (1932): pp. 194–98.

Howard, C.P. "Linitis Plastica. A study of Ten Cases". *Quarterly Journal of Medicine* 26, New Series, vol. 2 (January, 1933): pp. 59–78.

Howard, C.P. "The Rheumatic Lung". *Annals of Internal Medicine* 7 (August, 1933): pp. 165–71.

Howard, C.P. "Address of the Retiring President: The Educational Value of the Medical Society". *Bulletin of the Montreal Medico-Chirurgical Society* 3 (1935): pp. 52–55.

Howard, C. P. "The Diagnosis and Treatment of Malignant Hypertension". *Canadian Medical Association Journal* 32 (June, 1935): pp. 621–24.

Howard, C.P. "A Case of Early Scleroderma with Calcinosis." *Transactions of the Association of American Physicians* 50 (1935): pp. 88–91.

Howard, C.P. and Rhea, L.J. "A Case of Simmonds' Disease Due to a Primary Tumor of Rathke's Pouch, Observed Over a Period of Twelve Years". *International Clinics* 1 (1936): pp. 1–16.

Howard, C.P. "Scleroderma With Calcinosis". *Canadian Medical Association Journal* 37 (August, 1937): pp. 124–33.

Howard, C.P., Mills, E.S. and Townsend, S. R. "Paroxysmal Hemoglobinuria". *American Journal of the Medical Sciences* 196 (December, 1938): pp. 792–96.

Dates of Communications from Grace and William Osler with Citations to Cushing: *Life of Sir William Osler*

All communications are letters, unless otherwise indicated (in parentheses).

The Marjorie (Howard) Futcher collection consists of 94 communications. All express the sentiments of a parent devoted to a daughter, but the 55 listed also contain information relevant to the activities of Sir William, Lady Osler, Revere Osler or Campbell Howard.

1890
6/21 W.O. to CPH (illustrated post card)

1897
9/16 W.O. to CPH[1]

1901
6/11 W.O. to CPH; 8/21 W.O. to CPH[2]; 9/27 W.O. to CPH

1904
7/13 W.O. to CPH

1905
3/23 W.O. to CPH (signature written by secretary); 5/8 W.O. to CPH; 6/2 W.O. to CPH[3]; 7/14 W.O. to CPH; 7/22 W.O. to CPH; 8/3 W.O. to CPH; 8/13 W.O. to CPH; 8/24 W.O. to CPH; 9/18 W.O. to CPH; 10/21 W.O. to CPH (post card); 10/29 Grace O., Marjorie Howard, and W.O. to CPH[4]; 11/30 W.O., Marjorie H., E.Y.D. to CPH (post card)[5]; 12/13 W.O. to CPH

1906
2/21 W.O. to CPH (post card); 3/16 W.O. to Marjorie H.; 4/3 W.O. to CPH; 4/19 W.O. to CPH; 5/21 W.O. to CPH; 6/12 W.O. to CPH; 6/16 W.O. to CPH (post card); 6/29 W.O. to CPH; 7/11 W.O. to CPH (signature written by secretary); 10/19 W.O. to Marjorie H.; 10/25 W.O. to CPH

1907

1/16 W.O. to Marjorie H.; 1/31 W.O. to CPH; 2/15 W.O. to Principal Peterson[6]; 3/21 W.O. to Muriel Eberts; 4/17 W.O. to CPH; 5/11 W.O. to Marjorie H.; 5/20 W.O. to CPH (post card); 6/21 W.O. to CPH[7]; 8/2 W.O. to Marjorie H.; 10/7 W.O. to CPH[8]

1908

1/17 W.O. to CPH; 3/20 W.O. to Marjorie H.; 12/16 W.O. to CPH (post card)

1909

3/23 W.O. to CPH (illustrated post card); 5/31 W.O. to Marjorie H.; 7/2 W.O. to CPH (post card); 11/8 W.O. to Marjorie H.

1910

1/9 W.O. to Marjorie H. Futcher; 1/13 W.O. to CPH; 1/25 W.O. to Marjorie F. (post card); 4/3 W.O. to Marjorie F.; 4/20 W.O. to Marjorie F.; 4/25 W.O. to CPH; 7/28 W.O. to Principal Peterson[9]; 8/3 W.O. to Marjorie F.; 8/8 W.O. to CPH; 9/6 W.O. to CPH; 9/14 W.O. to Marjorie F.; 9/17 W.O. to CPH; 10/8 W.O. to CPH; 10/16 W.O. to Marjorie F.; 10/20 W.O. to CPH[10]; 11/11 W.O. to Marjorie F.; 11/24 W.O. to CPH; 12/16 W.O. to Marjorie F.

1911

1/4 W.O. to Marjorie F.; 1/15 W.O. to Marjorie F.; 2/10 W.O. to CPH (illustrated post card, Cairo); 2/13 W.O. to CPH (illustrated post card, Cairo); 2/20 W.O. to Marjorie F.; 2/28 W.O. to CPH (illustrated post card, Luxor); 3/3 W.O. to CPH (illustrated post card, Aswan (Karnak)); 3/28 W.O. to CPH; 4/11 W.O. to Marjorie F.; 5/3 W.O. to CPH; 5/11 W.O. to Principal Peterson[11]; 5/23 W.O. to CPH; 6/21 W.O. to Marjorie F.; 7/1 W.O. to CPH; 8/10 W.O. to Marjorie F.; 8/21 W.O. to CPH (enclosing Revere's ink sketches); 8/23 W.O. to CPH (telegram); 8/31 W.O. to Marjorie F.; 9/20 W.O. to CPH; 10/7 W.O. to Marjorie F.; 10/13 W.O. to CPH[12]; 12/15 W.O. to Marjorie F.

1912

1/8 Grace Osler to Principal Peterson[13]; 1/21 W.O. to Marjorie F.; 4/14 W.O. to CPH (post card); 4/28 W.O. to Marjorie F.; 7/17 W.O. to CPH; 8/14 W.O. to Marjorie F.; 12/10 W.O. to Marjorie F.; 12/12 W.O. to CPH (post card)

1913

1/23 W.O. to Marjorie F.; 4/13 W.O. to Marjorie F.; 4/27 W.O. to Marjorie F.; 5/3 W.O. to Marjorie F.; 5/9 W.O. to Marjorie F.; 5/24 W.O. to Marjorie F. (post card); 6/13 W.O. to Ottilie Howard (post card with photograph of W.O. and Group); 8/1 W.O. to Marjorie F.; 12/26 W.O. to Marjorie F.

1914

1/15 W.O. to Marjorie F.; 1/30 W.O. to CPH; 2/20 W.O. to CPH; 3/12 W.O. to CPH; 10/10 W.O. to Marjorie F.

1915
4/23 W.O. to Marjorie F.; 6/29 W.O. to Marjorie F.; 8/14 W.O. to CPH; 9/6 W.O. to CPH; 9/17 W.O. to CPH; 11/15 W.O. to Principal Peterson[14]; 11/18 W.O. to CPH; 12/17 W.O. to CPH

1916
1/15 W.O. to Prof. A. S. Warthin; 2/4 W.O. to Ottilie Howard; 3/8 W.O. and Grace Osler to Marjorie F.; 11/2 W.O. to Marjorie and Tom Futcher; 12/4 W.O. to CPH (enclosure to daughter Muriel is missing); 12/8 W.O. to Marjorie F.

1917
3/1 W.O. to Ottilie H.; 3/1 W.O. to CPH; 3/9 W.O. to Marjorie F.; 8/31 W.O. to CPH & Ottilie H[15]; 8/31 W.O. to Marjorie F.; 11/28 W.O. to Bruce F.; 12/4 W.O. to Marjorie F.; 12/4 W.O. to CPH[16]; 12/4 W.O. to Palmer Howard[17]

1918
2/14 W.O. to CPH; 4/6 W.O. to Marjorie F.; 9/27 Grace O. to Mrs. H.P. Wright[18]; 11/12 W.O. to Marjorie & Tom F.; 12/14 W.O. to Marjorie F.

1919
2/16 W.O. to Marjorie F.; 7/16 W.O. to CPH; 7/17 W.O. to CPH; 9/8 W.O. to CPH; 11/1 W.O. & Grace O. to CPH; 11/5 W.O. to Marjorie F.; 11/25 W.O. to CPH[19]

1. Cushing, *Life*, I, p. 459
2. Cushing, *Life*, I, p. 563–64
3. Cushing, *Life*, II, p. 5
4. Cushing, *Life*, II, 26 (incomplete)
5. E.Y.D. are the initials of Osler's alias, Egerton Y. Davis, Jr.
6. McGill U. Archives
7. Cushing, *Life*, II, p. 95
8. Cushing, *Life*, II, p. 103 (a few phrases)
9. McGill U. Archives
10. Cushing, *Life*, II, p. 244
11. McGill U. Archives
12. Cushing, *Life*, II, p. 297 (a few phrases)
13. McGill U. Archives
14. McGill U. Archives
15. Cushing, *Life*, II, p. 579 (with small changes)
16. Cushing, *Life*, II, p. 598 (under wrong date)
17. Cushing, *Life*, II, p. 587
18. Letter enclosed by Mrs. Wright to Ottilie H.
19. Cushing, *Life*, II, p. 679 (brief extracts)

Index

190   *Index*

192   *Index*

Louis, Pierre C. A., 44, 96, 117
Ludwig, Carl (1816–1895), 12

Macbride, Thomas H., 78
MacCallum, John Bruce, 96
MacCallum, William G., 24, 26
Macdonald, Sir William, 42
MacKenzie, Sir James, 84, 159
MacLean, George E., 50–51, 54–56
Macmichael, William, 43
MacNalty, Sir Arthur S., 95–96
Malloch, T. Archibald, 34, 40, 83, 95
Manson, Sir Patrick, 22
Marburg, William A., 39
Marie, Pierre, 40, 44
Martin, Charles F., 21, 43, 65, 92, 99
Matthews, Wilmot Love, 58
Matthews, Mrs. Wilmot L. (Annabel Margaret Osler, "Amo"), 58
Max-Müller, Rt. Hon. Friedrich (1823–1900), 28
Max-Müller, Mrs. F., 28
Mayo, Charles H., 91
Mayo, William J., 91
McClintock, John T., 98
McCrae, John, 20, 75, 77, 81, 87, 96, 115
McCrae, Thomas, 18, 20–21, 25–26, 28, 36, 43, 46, 63–64, 73–74, 91; served in Canadian Army, 73–74
McCrae, Mrs. T. (Amy Marion Gwyn), 46, 63
Meakins, John C., 84, 91–92
Medical News (Philadelphia), 6, 9
Meredith, Mrs. A.O.P. (Jean Wright), 27, 68, 77, 88
Meredith, Allen Pickton Osler, 88
Meredith, Mrs. Arthur (Isobel Marion Osler), 46, 88
Meredith, Frances Marion P. "Dinah" (Mrs. James O'Reilly), 46
Milburn, Edward Fairfax (Ned), 45, 67
Milton, John (1608–1674), 87
Mitchell, Silas Weir, 6, 8–10, 66, 96
Morgan, John, 8
Muirhead, Arnold, 15, 68
Murphy, Daniel D., 78
Murphy, John B., 76, 79, 84, 164
Müller, Friedrich von, 31, 35–37, 42–43

Nichols, Miss, see Smith, Nicola
Neusser, Edmond von, 39–40
Noorden, Carl H. von, 39–40

Oertel, Horst, 93
Olmstead, Ingersoll, 67
Osborne, Mrs. H. C. (Marian Georgina Francis), 58
Osler, Sir Edmund B., 58–61, 67, 87
Osler, Edward Revere (Dec. 28, 1895–July 30, 1917), nicknames, Isaac Walton, Ike, Tom, Tommy; godson of C.P. Howard, 34, 66; godfather of Bruce Futcher, 64, 86–87; godfather of Palmer Howard, 66, 86, social ac-

tivities, 17, 46, 57; interests, general, 16–17, 43; fishing, 20, 33, 43, 47, 56, 61, 63, 65, 84, 87; fine arts, 63–65, 69, 74; constructing, 64; literature, 69, 74–75, 81, 84, 86, 87; education at Winchester College, 16, 46–47, 63; at Oxford University, 72, 74–75; World War I service, Officers' Training Corps, 72, 74; No. 3 Canadian General Hospital, 75–77, 81; British Army Artillery, 81–86; mortal wound, 84–86; memorial gifts to godsons, 86–87; to Johns Hopkins University, Tudor & Stuart Club, 87
Osler, Rev. Featherstone Lake, 1–2, 158
Osler, Mrs. F. L. (Ellen Free Pickton), 1–2, 36
Osler, Lady (Grace Linzee Revere), 10–12, 14–16, 20, 22, 28–30, 33–34, 36–39, 44–47, 55–59, 61–65, 68, 72–75, 77, 81, 83–89, 93–96; married W. Osler, 14–15; personal character, 15, 72–73, 85–86; presented at Court, 61–62; illnesses, 15, 68–69; death, 15, will, 34, 68
Osler, Sir William (July 12, 1849–December 29, 1919:
Biography:
birth and childhood, 1; education, at Weston and Toronto, 1–2, 45; at McGill University, 2–3; postgraduate years abroad, 3–4; faculty appointments at McGill University and Montreal General Hospital, 4–7; teaching students at hospital bedside, 6, 9–10, 17, 74; Clinical Professor of Medicine, University of Pennsylvania, 8–10; attendance at death of Palmer Howard and continued contacts with Howard family, 10–12; Professor of Medicine, Johns Hopkins University and Physician-in-Chief of the Hospital, 10, 12–26; innovation of medical residency, 13; writing textbook, 14; marriage, 14–15; delight over his son Revere, 16, *et seq.;* influence on resident staff, including Campbell Howard, 18–21; trip to Britain and offer of Chair at Oxford, 21–22; farewell addresses in America, additions to *Aequanimitas,* 22–24; revision of textbook before departure in May, 1905, 24–26, 28; activities as Regius Professor of Medicine, Oxford University, 29–34; presentation of Harveian Oration, 38; offer of Presidency, University of Toronto, 39; advice regarding McGill Medical School, see Peterson, Sir William, and McGill; marriage of Marjorie Howard, 46; encouragement to Campbell Howard on appointment to Iowa, 55–57; godfather

14th.II.16

13, NORHAM GARDENS,
OXFORD.

Dear Campbell,

It was a sad business about poor Jack McCrae – pneumonia & meningitis. He had had sharp attacks of asthma, & had not had a good winter but he had stuck at it, & had just been apt. Consultant to the 1st. army. Birkett has gone back – wonderfully well – no rocks in bladder or pelvis

We keep much the same – house full all the time, & so many going & coming that we have not (fortunately) much time to think. Cleveland continue full of interest. The Heart Hospital has been moved to Colchester so I cannot go so often.

Mrs Wright & the girls are so well. Phoebe home on leave. How I wish you were all over here again. We miss the darlings so much. How splendidly they are growing. Love them well. Arthur Howard – better –

Love to O. & your dear self.

Yours

Ever W. O.